THE CONDITIONING HANDBOOK

The Conditioning Handbook: Getting in Top Shape

© 2006 IronMind Enterprises, Inc.

Cataloguing in Publication Data
Jones, Brian—
The conditioning handbook: getting in top shape
1. Fitness and health   2. Weightlifting   I. Title
2006 796.41 2006939185
ISBN 0-926888-14-5

Book cover and design by Tony Agpoon, Sausalito, California

Photo credits: Joshua Brown, Chris Heflin, Brian Jones, Tracy Wright

Models: Alan Browning, Olivia Eldridge, Victoria Graham, Jamie Hale, Chris Heflin, Brian Jones, Ryan Jones, Michael O'Donnell, Brian Ray, Tracy Wright

Published in the United States of America
IronMind Enterprises, Inc., P.O. Box 1228, Nevada City, CA 95959

Printed in the U.S.A. First Edition
10 9 8 7 6 5 4 3

THE CONDITIONING HANDBOOK

GETTING IN TOP SHAPE

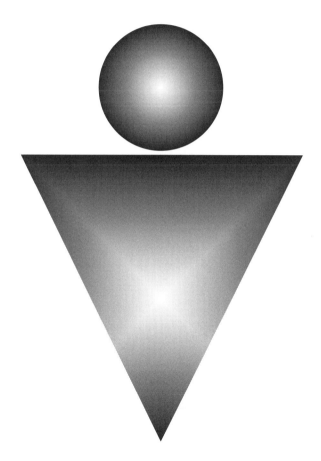

BRIAN JONES, M.S.

IronMind Enterprises, Inc.
Nevada City, California

This book is dedicated to my parents, Lester and Beth.
Without their love and support, it would not have been possible.

Other IronMind Enterprises Publications

SUPER SQUATS: How to Gain 30 Pounds of Muscle in 6 Weeks by Randall J. Strossen, Ph.D.

The Complete Keys to Progress by John McCallum, edited by Randall J. Strossen, Ph.D.

Mastery of Hand Strength by John Brookfield

IronMind: Stronger Minds, Stronger Bodies by Randall J. Strossen, Ph.D.

MILO: A Journal for Serious Strength Athletes, Randall J. Strossen, Ph.D., Publisher and Editor-in-chief

Powerlifting Basics, Texas-style: The Adventures of Lope Delk by Paul Kelso

Of Stones and Strength by Steve Jeck and Peter Martin

Sons of Samson, Volume 2 Profiles by David Webster

Rock Iron Steel: The Book of Strength by Steve Justa

Paul Anderson: The Mightiest Minister by Randall J. Strossen, Ph.D.

Louis Cyr: Amazing Canadian by Ben Weider, CM

Training with Cables for Strength by John Brookfield

The Grip Master's Manual by John Brookfield

Captains of Crush® Grippers: What They Are and How to Close Them by Randall J. Strossen, Ph.D., J. B. Kinney, and Nathan Holle

Winning Ways: How to Succeed In the Gym and Out by Randall J. Strossen, Ph.D.

The Complete Sandbag Training Course by Brian Jones

Bodyweight Exercises for Extraordinary Strength by Brad Johnson

To order additional copies of *The Conditioning Handbook: Getting in Top Shape* or for a catalog of IronMind Enterprises, Inc. publications and products, please contact:

IronMind Enterprises, Inc.
P.O. Box 1228
Nevada City, CA 95959 USA
tel: (530) 272-3579
fax: (530) 272-3095
website: www.ironmind.com
e-mail: sales@ironmind.com

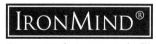

Stronger Minds, Stronger Bodies™

About the Author

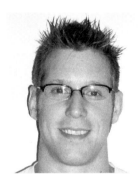

Brian Jones has an MS in exercise physiology and is a doctoral candidate at the University of Kentucky. He has been involved in strength and conditioning for many years and has trained athletes in a variety of sports from the high school to professional level. A judo and Brazilian jiujitsu instructor, Brian is especially interested in strength and conditioning as it applies to competitive fighters. Brian is the author of the popular *Complete Sandbag Training Course*, which has made sandbag training a staple in many strength and conditioning programs.

Acknowledgements

Thanks to Michael O'Donnell at Four Seasons Martial Arts, Mark Dickinson at Lexington Athletic Club, and Jamie Hale at Total Body Fitness for the use of their equipment and facilities.

Table of Contents

Introduction

Browse the sports and fitness section of any bookstore and you'll see numerous books on conditioning and endurance training. Every college exercise physiology textbook also usually has a few chapters devoted to cardio-respiratory exercise. By and large these books do a good job of covering the basics of how the body responds and adapts to exercise. However, when it comes to showing you the practical aspects of setting up an endurance program, they fall short. All they usually suggest is 30 to 45 minutes of continuous low- to moderate-intensity work at 65% to 75% of heart rate max, on the track or the cardio machine of your choice.

If you look around your gym, you'll see that this is just what people are doing, plodding along at a comfortable pace on the latest high-tech gizmo like hamsters on wheels, all the while listening to music, watching movies on the cardio theatre, or talking on their cell phones to distract them from their boring workouts. If this behavior were limited to a few people training under doctors' orders, it would not be of concern. What is bothersome is that this type of endurance work is used so frequently by strength athletes, fighters, and others who are training for performance. After spending hours grunting, straining, and bleeding in a cloud of ammonia and liniment, they crank out their half hour of light cycling because they feel they need to.

One has to ask, "Is this the ONLY way to get in shape?" Aren't there types of training that will burn fat and build endurance other than the dreaded long, slow, distance workouts? Yes, there are. *There are so many alternative ways to do endurance work you could fill a book . . . and in fact, you are reading it right now*. Personally, I can't stand logging in hours on a treadmill, and since I do not run marathons or even 10Ks, I don't want to jog whenever I need to build my endurance, nor do I want to cycle endless miles at an easy pace while I watch reruns on TV. I'm happy to tell all the lifters, fighters, and fitness enthusiasts that such an opinion has not doomed me to a life of low aerobic and anaerobic endurance. Rather it has made me a bit more resourceful when planning my workouts.

There is little that is truly new in the world of strength and conditioning. Chances are that anything you believe you invented was a staple in someone's training 50 years ago. Therefore I consider this book a work of synthesis. I present it to you as a collection of training information and ideas gathered from formal education, experience as an athlete and coach, my reading, conversations with other coaches, and other sources too numerous to mention. I have, of course, added many of my own ideas and training programs, but I must give credit to all of my influences.

I wrote this book for everyone who wants to build endurance without necessarily training like an endurance athlete. It is for powerlifters, weightlifters, strongmen, wrestlers, football players, judoka, boxers, and mixed martial artists. It is written for everyone who prefers to be in the moment during a workout, focusing on the next rep or exercise rather than doing what they can to be somewhere, anywhere else than training. If you are reading this book now it was most likely written just for you.

The Conditioning Handbook: Getting in Top Shape is a comprehensive guide to conditioning. Most training books devote only a chapter or two to conditioning work and thus contain only a few general concepts. Readers are left wondering how to put these general concepts into practice. *The Conditioning Handbook: Getting in Top Shape* covers conditioning from the ground up. It lays a foundation with the physiology of training adaptations and general concepts relevant to physical training. It then builds on the concepts by exploring how they are applied in the day-to-day workout environment. Numerous workout formats, templates, exercise modalities, and example workouts fill in the gaps left by other books and provide a complete source of conditioning information for the reader.

I hope *The Conditioning Handbook: Getting in Top Shape* inspires you to achieve a high level of endurance—with enjoyment—in your training.

Abbreviations

In the interest of space, I use several abbreviations when referring to training or writing workouts:

BB – barbell
DB – dumbbell
KB – kettlebell
MB – medicine ball
SB – stability ball (or Swiss ball)
IC – Indian club
bwt – bodyweight
1RM – one-rep maximum
> – greater than
< – less than

Sets and repetition schemes are written as sets x reps (load), so 3 x 10 (75%) means 3 sets of 10 repetitions at 75% of your one-rep maximum (1RM). Where relevant, rest intervals will be given after the load.

CHAPTER 1

PHYSIOLOGY OF CONDITIONING

This section of the book covers the essentials of exercise physiology as they apply to conditioning. While this material may not be as exciting as the how-to of program design and exercise technique, it will dramatically enhance your ability to design effective conditioning programs. Armed with this information, you will also be better able to critically analyze programs written by others. Many people claim to have all the answers when it comes to physical training, and it is up to you to evaluate these recommendations from an informed standpoint. For some reason or another, coaches and athletes often feel that digging into the physiology of training is too difficult or a waste of time. As a result there are many supposed training gurus who know much more about the inner workings of their cars and computers than their own bodies. Take some time to understand specifically how the body adapts to training. Don't shortchange yourself by skipping this section. Read it and use it both as a reference and a starting point for further research.

Some Basic Definitions

GPP vs. SPP Training

The terms GPP and SPP get tossed around a lot during most discussions of strength and conditioning. GPP stands for *general physical preparation* and is often referred to as work capacity. GPP does not refer to a specific physiological attribute but is a composite of many different attributes. A useful way to think of GPP is as the base of the athletic training pyramid. It is a foundation of fitness that you will build on. If you have an acceptable level of GPP, you will be able to perform a wide variety of tasks. General physical training involves a varied training routine that simultaneously builds aerobic and anaerobic endurance, local muscular endurance, strength, power, and flexibility. Without GPP, you will not be able to tolerate the training loads and volumes necessary for optimal performance in your given sport. Many lifters neglect GPP training, taking very long rests between sets and never doing any other conditioning work. They will tell you that a person needs 5-minute rest intervals and that any extra conditioning will interfere with muscle or strength gains. This simply isn't true. It is just an excuse to cover up a lack of fitness and desire to condition themselves. Research has shown that just 1 minute's rest is enough time for most people to repeat a 1RM lift.

GPP training is ideal for young trainees. Children should build a wide range of athletic skills during development, only specializing or training very heavily once they have finished growing. Unfortunately, physical education in American schools is often neglected and kids have spent increasing amounts of free time playing video games or watching television. Adults with no history of sports or physically active recreation and with current sedentary lifestyles are going to need a longer GPP build-up phase.

GPP training methods include:

- doing full-body circuit training routines
- learning to control one's bodyweight using bodyweight exercises
- evening up muscular imbalances
- building general athleticism through basic functional movements, such as running, jumping, or tumbling
- developing range of motion and flexibility throughout the body
- performing corrective exercises necessary to prevent injury
- learning proper exercise technique using lighter loads
- building strength and endurance in the trunk or core muscles
- developing an aerobic base
- using a variety of exercise modes for all-around muscular development

SPP stands for *specific physical preparation* and is synonymous with sport-specific training. After establishing a GPP base, each athlete must develop a training schedule that maintains general fitness levels while emphasizing those attributes most relevant to his or her sport. Typically SPP training utilizes more advanced methods of training which may not be appropriate or safe for trainees without a proper fitness base. The exact SPP methods vary widely among sports.

One of the drawbacks to the functional training movement is that some coaches and trainees do not take the time to develop GPP before moving into SPP training. This oversight causes their training programs to fall short or cause injuries. Specific training must always build on a foundation of general fitness. There is no point in worrying about adding weight to the bar in the bench press if you can't do a decent set of push-ups or do a single pull-up. There is also little to be gained by mimicking sporting movements with an 8-pound dumbbell while standing on a Swiss ball if you haven't built a minimal degree of strength on the basic lifts. Unfortunately both of these situations are common, especially with high school athletes. Always ensure a solid foundation before using more advanced training methods.

SPP training methods are more advanced and include:

- full-body and/or split training routines
- advanced bodyweight and gymnastic exercises
- high-load, low-repetition exercises to develop limit strength
- intense hypertrophy training methods, such as forced repetitions, cheat repetitions, or drop sets
- partial movements and functional isometrics
- plyometrics and complex training
- high-intensity interval training
- planned over-reaching, super-compensation, and peaking schedules

When Is GPP Sufficient?

There are no hard and fast rules for deciding when you or your athletes have acceptable GPP and can begin using more specific training methods. You must come up with some sort of testing battery that addresses different fitness attributes. The exact tests used and the minimally acceptable scores will vary depending on the coach, athlete, and sports in question. Here are some suggested minimal scores that I use with my athletes:

	Men	Women
Bodyweight control		
push-ups	20 reps	5 reps
pull-ups	5 reps	1 rep (or 5 recline rows)
bodyweight squats	50 reps	50 reps
sit-ups	40 reps in 60 sec.	40 reps in 60 sec.
Basic strength		
bench press	1.0 x bwt.	0.5 x bwt.
squat	1.25 x bwt.	1 x bwt.
deadlift	1.25 x bwt.	1 x bwt.
power clean	0.75 x bwt.	0.5 x bwt.
Strength endurance		
20-rep barbell squat	50% 1RM	50% 1RM
20-rep bench press	60% 1RM	60% 1RM
20-rep DB/KB 1-arm snatch	0.20 x bwt.	0.10 x bwt.
Aerobic base endurance		
timed mile run	10 min.	10 min.
5K run	30 min.	30 min.

Athletes who meet most, but not all, standards may progress to more specific training while performing work designed to improve their weaknesses. You can do additional sets, workouts, or alternative exercises for your underdeveloped attributes while doing more advanced work for your strong areas. If you are larger or heavier, some of these bodyweight movements and percentages may take longer to achieve or may need to be adjusted downward. However, don't assume that just because you are large you shouldn't be able to control your bodyweight. Work at it consistently rather than giving up and using your size as an excuse. The goal with testing GPP is to add an objective measure to your decisions about training. Any numbers must be interpreted in light of what you know about your unique situation.

GPP, SPP, and Seasonal Periodization

If you play a sport that is organized into seasons or if you have designated a particular time of the year as a competition period, you will need to fluctuate between emphasizing GPP and SPP methods depending on where you are in the competition cycle. In the off-season, when there are no practice sessions or they are not as demanding, this is the time to work more on GPP. Your strength and conditioning workouts can be higher volume and intensity, and you can develop general strength, power, athleticism, and if desired, mass. Conditioning workouts should focus on maintaining a basic level of aerobic and anaerobic endurance. The off-season is the best time to experiment with new training methods and learn new lifting techniques. Focus on building many attributes simultaneously and enhancing GPP. Obviously there will be a thread of SPP running throughout off-season workouts. The degree of specific training is determined by how well you have prepared in previous seasons.

In the pre-season, your sport's practices will take up most of your energy. Consequently you must lower the volume of your strength and conditioning work. Most of the training during this phase will be SPP. All conditioning activities that are not directly related to your sport should be dropped. Pre-season training builds on the fitness you developed in the off-season. Many athletes neglect strength and conditioning work in the off-season, thereby losing valuable work capacity. They struggle through pre-season workouts and are at a much greater risk of injury. It is no coincidence that they are usually the same athletes who never seem to live up to their potential.

During the competitive season, the focus is on maintaining your fitness levels. Due to the demands of practices and games, the volume and intensity of the strength and conditioning workouts must drop dramatically. Workouts should consist entirely of SPP methods.

A final phase that many athletes neglect is a post-season active recovery phase. The rigors of a yearly training cycle can take their toll on you physically and mentally. A 2- to 4-week break from organized training can do wonders for your mind and body. You can maintain your fitness levels during this time with recreational games, light jogging, hiking, or anything else that is unrelated to your sport.

Bioenergetics

All physical activity requires energy. However, the means by which the energy is provided differs according to the type of activity performed. In exercise physiology, the study of how the body produces energy is called bioenergetics. Several distinct energy pathways are used to produce the ATP that serves as cellular fuel. Each pathway uses a unique combination of structures and enzymes and produces energy in different amounts and at different rates. These pathways also use different fuel sources. All of them run continuously during any activity but their relative importance to energy production differs from activity to activity. The adaptations resulting from stressing a particular energy pathway are specific to that pathway. For this reason, your training must mimic the activity you are training for very closely if it is to have much impact on performance.

ATP

The molecule ATP (adenosine triphosphate) is the energy currency of the human body. It powers every action you perform, from muscular contractions to the basic metabolic processes that keep you alive. Your body needs ATP to maintain homeostasis or the dynamic balance of your bodily systems. Food provides the raw materials from which ATP is produced. The muscles keep a small amount of ATP on hand for immediate use. The rest of the ATP provided is either resynthesized by the phosphagen system, or it is produced by the breakdown of blood sugar (glucose) and sugar stored in the muscles and liver (glycogen), by the glycolytic system; by fatty acids stored in adipose tissue, by the oxidative system; or by proteins from muscle tissue.

Phosphagen System

The body stores a small amount of ATP and a substance called creatine phosphate (CP) within skeletal muscle. Together these form the phosphagen system and are responsible for supplying quick energy for short duration activities. Stored ATP is broken down into another molecule called ADP, which releases energy to power activity. In order to maintain energy production, CP rapidly converts ADP back to ATP using an enzyme called creatine kinase. This process does not require oxygen and is therefore anaerobic. The phosphagen system also does not produce lactic acid as a by-product like the other anaerobic system, glycolysis. However, the muscles' supply of CP is also limited so this process can only provide energy for activities lasting 3 seconds or less, like:

- heavy singles (e.g., deadlift, bench press, snatch)
- short sprints (e.g., 40-yd. or 100-yd. dash)
- long jumps or broad jumps
- javelin or hammer throws and shot puts

Creatine supplements influence the activity of the phosphagen system by increasing the stores of CP within the muscles. With additional CP, this system can produce more energy before the body must resort to glycolysis.

Glycolytic System

The second method used to produce energy is through the breakdown of free sugar (glucose) or stored sugar (glycogen). This process is called glycolysis and the system is known as the glycolytic system. Intense activities of 4 to 50 seconds in duration rely primarily on this system. In glycolysis, glucose molecules are quickly broken down to produce ATP and lactic acid by a process that does not require oxygen. Glucose sources in the body include circulating blood glucose as well as glycogen stores in skeletal muscle and in the liver. The downside to glycolysis is that it forms lactic acid, a substance that is toxic to the body. As lactic acid levels rise, the acidity of the blood increases, causing that familiar weakness, burning, and nausea common during high-intensity work.

The glycolytic system is the predominant energy pathway during:

- 100 to 800 m sprints
- fighting exchanges within a boxing or wrestling match
- a football play
- a tennis volley

Oxidative System

The final energy producing system is the oxidative (aerobic) system. It produces the energy to power long-duration (greater than 2 minutes), lower-intensity activity such as distance runs. Products produced by the glycolytic system along with circulating fatty acids and stored fat are used to produce large amounts of ATP. Under most circumstances, fuel availability does not limit the oxidative system as it does in the phosphagen system: most people have ample amounts of stored body fat. It also does not produce performance limiting by-products like the lactic acid of glycolysis. Most of the energy for normal daily activities is produced by this system. The drawback to the oxidative system is that it takes more time to produce ATP, so when the activity is quick or intense it cannot keep up and the anaerobic systems have to take up the slack.

The oxidative system provides energy for:

- a 1-mile to marathon distance run
- long swims or cycling
- jogging down the field in soccer

VO2 Max

In exercise physiology the primary measure used for quantifying endurance capacity is VO2 max. VO2 max is defined as your body's maximal ability to take in and use oxygen. It depends on a number of different factors. Two primary factors determine VO2 max: maximal cardiac output and oxygen extraction.

Maximal cardiac output is the ability of the heart to pump blood throughout the body. The higher the cardiac output, the more oxygenated blood is delivered to working muscles. It is determined by maximal heart rate (HR) and maximal stroke volume (SV), or the amount of blood pumped during each beat. The formula, then, is:

$$max\ cardiac\ output = HR\ max * SV\ max$$

Maximal heart rate is a fixed value that changes little with training. However, stroke volume can be altered by conditioning work. With training, the chamber volume of your left ventricle increases to accommodate more blood. This adaptation is primarily a result of longer duration or distance endurance training. Lifting and high-intensity endurance work also increase the strength of the cardiac muscle. Harder contractions pump out more of the blood in the heart with each beat. These two factors combine to increase stroke volume.

The second main factor in VO2 max is oxygen extraction, or how much of the oxygen in the blood is taken up by working muscles. After all, getting oxygen to the muscles does little good if the muscles can't use it. Extraction is measured by finding the difference between the oxygen content of arterial blood (blood going from the heart) and that of venous blood (blood returning to the heart). Oxygen extraction increases dramatically with endurance training, as the muscle has a greater number of mitochondria and capillaries that make it more efficient at removing and using oxygen.

In the laboratory, VO2 max is a measure of exercise intensity. Intensities of 100% VO2 max and below represent primarily aerobic or oxidative energy production, while those in excess of 100% represent more of a reliance on anaerobic energy production.

Lactate Threshold

Lactic acid (or lactate) is a by-product of the breakdown of sugar by anaerobic glycolysis. Glycolytic metabolism occurs all the time, not just during intense exercise. This means that you are always producing a small amount of lactic acid, even at rest. The lactic acid has almost no effect on blood pH because your body is able to buffer and metabolize it as quickly as it is produced. Blood lactate levels at any given time, then, represent a balance between the rate of production and the rate of clearance. Your body's lactic acid clearance system works well enough that even during light- to moderate-intensity exercise there will be very little change in blood acidity. As intensity climbs further, there will be a point at which production exceeds clearance capacity and the pH of your blood drops substantially. This is known as the lactate threshold and it occurs in most people at around 60 to 70% of VO2 max.

Lactic acid accumulation is a major factor in fatigue. High levels cause pain and nausea and can interfere with muscle contraction. You can work at intensities below the lactate threshold for extended periods, but performance above threshold cannot be maintained for long. Conditioning training pushes the lactate threshold higher by decreasing production and increasing clearance ability. This allows you to push harder for a longer period than before, thus enhancing performance.

Causes of Fatigue

Fatigue is the inability to maintain the required force or work output in some activity. In other words, it is the point when you get tired and can no longer keep up the pace or have to stop. Thus the ultimate goal of conditioning is to develop your fatigue resistance, your ability to perform at a higher level for a longer duration. All fatigue is not the same. The underlying mechanisms that cause you to fatigue differ according to type of activity.

The following section discusses the physiological factors limiting different types of exercise performances.

Very short (< 10 sec.)

Maximal efforts of 10 seconds or less require you to produce a lot of energy very quickly. Your ability to recruit fast twitch (type II) motor units is a major factor limiting performances of this duration. Fast twitch motor units are composed of muscle fibers that can produce high force quickly. The downside is that they are not very energy efficient, they fatigue rapidly, and they produce more lactic acid than slow twitch fibers. Most of the energy for activities of 10 seconds or less is provided by the phosphagen system, with some coming from anaerobic glycolysis.

Thus, the limiting factors in very short efforts are:

- motivation and type II motor unit recruitment
- skill in the movement
- amount of stored ATP and CP in skeletal muscle

Short (10–180 sec.)

Activities involving all-out efforts of 10 to 180 seconds use different pathways depending on where in this range they fall. At the low end, about 70% of the energy is produced anaerobically by a combination of the phosphagen and glycolytic systems. At the other end (around 3 minutes), as much as 60% of the energy is produced aerobically by oxidative pathways. Anaerobic pathways produce energy quickly but create lactic acid as a by-product. Lactic acid decreases blood pH, causing discomfort and interfering with the contractile mechanisms within the muscle.

The limiting factors in short activities, then, are:

- amount of stored ATP and CP in skeletal muscle: the longer the phosphagen system can supply energy, the less lactic acid is produced
- lactic acid buffering capacity
- ability to switch to oxidative energy production sooner
- VO2 max

Medium (3–20 min.)

As the time increases from 3 to 20 minutes, you rely increasingly on aerobic energy sources. In fact, after 20 minutes of all-out activity, as much as 90% of the energy comes from the oxidative pathway. Maximal efforts of this duration usually involve your working at greater than 90% VO2 max; thus oxidative capacity is the primary determinant in performance. However, other factors are involved as well. Lactic acid build-up from the glycolytic pathway hinders performance, so the sooner you can switch to oxidative metabolism, the less fatigue you will accumulate. Endurance training will cause you to switch to oxidative pathways sooner and thus produce less lactic acid for a given exercise duration. Also your ability to effectively buffer the lactic acid that is produced will help prevent increases in blood acidity and its negative effect on performance.

The limiting factors of medium-duration performances are:

- VO2 max
- ability to switch to oxidative energy production sooner
- lactic acid buffering capacity

Intermediate (21–60 min.)

During activities that last from 21 minutes to about one hour, the primary energy pathway is oxidative so VO2 max is a major factor in performance. However, at this duration, biomechanical factors become increasingly important. Any activity has an associated movement cost to maintain a given workload. The more efficient you are with your movements, the less energy you will burn to maintain a given work output. This is especially evident when switching your mode of exercise. For instance, if you run frequently, then you will be quite efficient with the movement. You will have an easy stride and minimal arm movement, and those muscles that are not directly involved will be relaxed. If you try to substitute your normal 30-minute run with an exercise that you aren't so proficient in, you'll get tired much faster. Your efficiency drops and it takes much more energy to maintain the pace. A final factor is lactate threshold. Staying under lactate threshold is important to prevent drops in blood pH from interfering with performance. A higher lactate threshold means you can maintain a faster pace.

The major limiting factors in intermediate-duration work are:

- VO2 max
- movement economy or efficiency
- lactate threshold

Long (1–4 hr.)

Extended workouts or long-distance endurance training relies almost exclusively on oxidative energy pathways. VO2 max is again important, but your maximal capacity is less important than the highest percentage of VO2 max you can maintain without crossing the lactate threshold. Movement economy is also a major factor in long duration exercise. Inefficient bio-mechanics or unfamiliar movements will require much more energy and cause greater fatigue. With activities requiring over an hour of continuous activity, fuel depletion and dehydration can become factors in fatigue. Your body stores sugar as glycogen in the muscles and liver. After about 90 minutes of continuous work, the supply can become exhausted. This depletion causes a dramatic decrease in your rate of energy production and a feeling of severe fatigue— what marathoners and other endurance athletes call "hitting the wall."

Long-duration activity also results in substantial water loss due to sweating. Dehydration causes an earlier onset of fatigue due to problems with cooling and a higher heart rate needed to compensate for dropping blood pressure. It is critical that water and easily digestible carbo-hydrates be consumed during the workout or competition.

The limiting factors in long-duration activity are:

- lactate threshold
- movement economy or efficiency
- VO2 max
- glycogen storage
- hydration status

Energy System Specificity of Training Adaptations

Specificity in training makes intuitive sense with strength training. For larger, stronger legs, lower-body training, like squats and deadlifts, is the key. Most of the strength and hypertrophy will occur in the trained muscles. But the specificity factor is equally important in conditioning. Just because 30 minutes at a moderate pace on the stair-climber machine gets you sweaty and out-of-breath does not mean that it will do anything for your sprinting or farmer's walk performance. The reason is that they activate different energy systems.

Stated simply, to train a particular energy system, you must choose conditioning methods that activate that system, as shown in the earlier discussion:

- train the phosphagen system using very short, high-intensity activities lasting only a few seconds
- train the glycolytic system with short, high-intensity activities lasting longer than 4 seconds but fewer than 60 seconds
- train the oxidative system with longer, low-intensity activities lasting in excess of 2 minutes

It is important to note, however, that the specificity principle does not mean that during a given activity, *only one* energy system is utilized. There will always be overlap in your training. During any activity all systems will be running; however the type of conditioning activity determines which of these systems will be the dominant energy producer and thus receives the greatest training effect.

Physiological Adaptations to Conditioning

Endurance adaptations can be divided into central and peripheral. Central adaptations affect the body as a whole and include such things as the capacity of the heart and lungs to supply blood to the working muscles as well as properties of the blood itself, like total volume and oxygen-carrying capacity. Peripheral adaptations are responses at the level of the skeletal muscles. These include the degree of concentrations of energy-producing enzymes, mitochondria, fuel storage, and blood supply. Both central and peripheral adaptations are required for increased performance.

Central adaptations – heart, lungs, and blood

- increased heart chamber volume – more blood pumped per beat to working muscles results in a lower heart rate at rest and during exercise

- increased heart muscle contractility – heart muscle contracts harder on each beat, pumping out more of the blood that is in the chamber; this is known as an increased ejection fraction

- increased endurance of ventilatory muscles – the accessory muscles that aid in maximal breathing rates become more resistant to fatigue

- increased hematocrit – the hemoglobin content of the blood increases so that it is able to carry more oxygen to, and carbon dioxide from, the cells

- increased acid-buffering capacity – your ability to buffer the lactic acid produced by glycolysis increases, resulting in less discomfort and fatigue

Peripheral adaptations – muscles and limbs

- increased intramuscular fuel storage – storage of ATP, CP, glycogen, and fatty acids within the muscles increases so that they are more readily available for fuel contraction

- increased mitochondrial density – the mitochondria are the cells' energy producers; training increases the amount of mitochondrial tissue and its associated enzymes

- increased capillary density – capillaries are tiny blood vessels required to bring oxygenated blood to working muscles and to remove metabolic waste products; a greater number of capillaries surrounding muscle fibers makes this process more efficient

- changes in energy-producing enzymes – the enzymes responsible for glycolysis and aerobic metabolism undergo changes in quality and/or structure so that more energy can be produced faster with less lactic acid build-up

To illustrate the effect of central and peripheral conditioning, let us take the example of two athletes, one who conditions primarily through running workouts and another whose workouts are mostly swimming. We will assume that each has a comparable workout schedule and similar central adaptation. Their hearts pump equally forcefully and move a lot of blood with each beat, and their lungs extract similar amounts of oxygen from the air and give off similar amounts of carbon dioxide. However, due to their particular training modes—one mostly runs and the other mostly swims, their peripheral adaptations will differ. For the swimmer, the specific muscles used in swimming will have developed peripheral adaptations, and for the runner it will be the running muscles. If the two were to switch workouts for a week, neither would likely be able to perform at the level of the other. This would be the case even if we assumed that both athletes were equally proficient in the techniques of running and swimming. Their lack of peripheral adaptations for the specific type of exercise would limit their performance: arm and leg muscles would cramp and burn long before their hearts and lungs were taxed.

This effect was shown experimentally in a study in which the subjects trained using one-leg-only cycling. At the end of the training program, the subjects' VO2 max went up but only when tested using the trained leg. VO2 max testing using the untrained leg showed no improvement. The enhanced capacity of the lungs and heart to get blood to the muscles did nothing because the muscles did not have the ability to use that oxygen. Conditioning work is very mode-specific, which means that if you are training for a sport, you must mimic the activities of your sport. It also means that if you want all-around development, you must use a wide variety of modalities.

Psychological Adaptations

Psychological adaptations, although often not discussed, are extremely important to conditioning. High-intensity or long-duration activities often become painful due to lactic acid build-up and other forms of fatigue. Developing a tolerance for this discomfort is part of increasing performance. Very few people are able to push themselves to their true physiological performance limits because the pain of fatigue convinces them to stop. Repeated conditioning sessions are a form of inoculation against the temptation to quit when the going gets tough. This resistance to giving up is the true meaning of *mind over matter*.

Despite all of the physiological literature dealing with the causes of fatigue in the human body, most fatigue is not physiological, but volitional. In other words, people decide to stop working. Due to ethics in human research, people cannot be forced to work harder than they choose. They work until they feel they can't go on anymore and quit, and that point is regarded as their max. Now raise the stakes and try it again. Most likely these same people could put their max performances to shame in a situation of real-life emergency when they, or their loved ones, were in danger. The elite can summon this type of effort on command. The ability to push yourself this hard develops with long-term serious training, just as with physiological mechanisms.

The point of this is not to suggest that anyone works out so hard that he or she drops dead. Rather, it is to illustrate how important the mind is in exercise performance. Strength of mind must be built just like strength of body, but it can only be built by persisting when all you want to do is quit. The need to train your mind is something to consider the next time you feel like dropping the last few sets or reps of your workout.

Body Recomposition

Certainly a lot of adaptation goes on inside the body as a result of conditioning training. However, the most visible effect is a decrease in stored body fat. Conditioning, particularly at higher intensities, burns an enormous number of calories. If your caloric intake doesn't increase, you will usually see noticeable reductions in body fat within the first month of conditioning. In addition to the aesthetic benefit, there are many health and performance reasons to stay lean.

Keeping body fat under 20% in men or 25% in women is associated with a much lower risk of most major diseases. All other things being equal, lean people have less heart disease, diabetes, and cancer than obese people do. Although you may not consider this a motivation to train if you're young, it will become increasingly important as you age. From a performance standpoint, think of extra body fat as a weight vest. Imagine going to work each day, training, and playing sports wearing an extra 20 or 30 pounds strapped to you. Think what a relief it would be to finally take that off. Body fat is metabolically inactive tissue. It has mass but does not perform work, thus increasing the energy requirement of movement. Your movements are less efficient and you fatigue much faster than you should. Subcutaneous body fat also acts as an insulator, holding in heat and making it harder for your body to cool itself.

You do need a certain amount of body fat for general health and padding. For athletes, a range of 8 to 10% for men and 12 to 15% for women is low enough. Dropping below this will cause both health and performance problems. Bodybuilders who get excessively lean for contests and photo shoots often have joint pain and skin that is painfully sensitive. Though excessively low body fat is not typically a problem, it can be if you do too much conditioning, have poor nutritional habits, or have an eating disorder.

Recent scientific research has found that high-intensity training may be more effective than the traditionally prescribed long-duration moderate-intensity work. There are two main reasons that this could be the case. First, as intensity increases, your body becomes less efficient. Decreased efficiency means that the energy cost of high-intensity work is much higher per unit time than low-intensity work. A short high-intensity workout may burn the same or more calories than a longer low-intensity session. The second reason is due to an increase in metabolic rate after the workout. The phenomenon is known as excess post-exercise oxygen consumption (EPOC). Following any exercise bout, there will be a period of increased oxygen uptake and elevated metabolic rate. High-intensity exercise causes a significantly greater and longer-lasting EPOC than low-intensity. Thus there may be a greater total caloric expenditure over the course of the day, especially if you do the training early in the morning.

CHAPTER 2

PROGRAMMING

Programming is putting together an effective training program using a combination of scientific principles and practical knowledge. Strength and conditioning are equal parts science and art. Exercise physiology research has established basic operating procedures for physical training. Overlooking or ignoring the knowledge provided by such research is a recipe for failure. Within the bounds of these training principles, however, there is much room for preference and creativity. This is where experience, both as coach and trainee, comes into play. You must experiment and find out which workout formats, exercises, sets, and repetition schemes work best for different goals. You must also determine when to schedule workouts and at what intensity and volume given your or your athletes' recovery capacity. Coaches training entire teams must find out how to best implement their training ideas in a group setting and how to balance the convenience of training uniformity with the necessity to accommodate individual needs among their athletes.

Hard Work

Before going any further you must understand the one immutable and absolute law governing all physical training and any other training you undertake. Simply stated:

input = output

Regardless of your particular training philosophy or the methods you choose to implement, you will only get out what you put in. No one has ever accomplished any meaningful physical transformation without hard work and persistence. The greatest coach, best training partners, and most proven program will do nothing for you unless you are prepared to work out regularly and give it everything you've got. Hard work doesn't mean just getting to the gym or half-heartedly going through the motions during a training session just to get finished. If this is your idea of training, you will never achieve your goals.

Workout time is workout time. It is not a time to socialize, flirt, or talk on your cell phone. You must make sacrifices. You must train even when it is inconvenient. You must push yourself out of your comfort zone time and time again.

Principles of Training

Overload

Your body constantly strives to maintain homeostasis. Homeostasis can be thought of as a dynamic balance wherein various physiological variables are maintained around a certain set point. Your body's homeostatic mechanisms act much like a thermostat to keep these variables from deviating too much from the desired points. In order to improve any physical attribute, including the previously discussed energy systems, you must overload that system or push it beyond the demands to which it has become accustomed. Overload is a form of stress that challenges your body's ability to maintain homeostasis. When stressed, your body undergoes acute responses, such as elevated body temperature, heart rate, and breathing, in an attempt to meet the challenge. Because this is taxing to your system and depletes fuel stores, the stress will be followed by a period of fatigue. However, if a period of rest and recovery is allowed following the stress, the body will undergo adaptations that will help it deal with that stress in the future. Thus, the formula for training can be summarized as:

stress + rest = progress

Recovery

Recovery refers to the rest portion of the above equation. Progress is not made during the workout, but rather in the time between workouts when your body is busy building muscle, strengthening connective tissue, increasing capillary density, and creating the enzymes that will boost your endurance. If recovery is compromised, then no progress will happen. What many trainees fail to realize is that proper recovery means more than just waiting a couple of days before the next workout or rotating body parts during the training week. It means eating the right foods, supplementing when necessary, getting an appropriate amount of sleep, and minimizing life stress to the extent possible. Your individual rate and capacity of recovery will to a large extent determine how hard and frequently you can train and still make progress. In addition to your genetics and lifestyle, your fitness level and age are major factors in recovery. As a rule, fitter and younger people recover faster from training stresses.

Progression

This principle is a function of the overload and recovery principles. If after applying stress and allowing for recovery you simply stopped training, your body would undergo a positive adaptation, maintain it for a short while, then lose it because it was not needed. In fact, this is what many people who fail to adhere to exercise programs do. They work out, get sore, and then lose motivation and never return to the gym. To maintain the adaptation and further increase your fitness, you must apply stress again following the recovery interval by sticking to an ongoing training program.

As your fitness increases, the overload stress must be increased to elicit further adaptations. In theory, progressive overload is linear, and the stress should be increased during each workout. In practice, however, it is not always that simple. During yearly, monthly, and weekly training cycles, there should be periods of varying intensity so that during some workouts you are training well under your ability, some just at your capacity, and some near your limits. What in theory is a linear development is in reality more of a sawtooth relationship. Progression is a "two steps forward, one step back" affair. This is especially true if you are already a well-trained athlete. With a properly designed program, there should always be steady upward trend in your performance. If this isn't the case you must reevaluate and change your program.

Specificity

Different types of training result in different physiological adaptations. This is the primary reason that different athletes must use different training methods to prepare for respective sports. A competitive lifter does not need the same degree of aerobic capacity as a distance runner. Likewise, the runner does not need to develop his or her limit strength to the same degree as the lifter. For optimal development of particular attributes such as strength, flexibility, or aerobic endurance, it is essential to utilize training modalities that stress the appropriate bodily structures and systems. This is the reason the earlier discussion of energy systems is so important for conditioning work. It is also important to realize that your body is an interconnected whole and that training one attribute will always have some effect on the others. Understanding these interconnections allows you to design efficient programs that build many attributes simultaneously.

The specificity principle has three primary dimensions: 1) energy pathways, 2) muscle groups, and 3) movement patterns. Attention to all of them will ensure the greatest amount of performance carryover to the activity you're training for.

Individuality

We are all human and therefore share a common physiology. This fact allows generalizations to be made regarding our responses to exercise. However, there can be a great deal of inter-individual variation with regard to training. Differences can include the speed of adaptation to exercise, tolerance of exercise loads and volumes, responses to particular modes of training, and ultimate capacity for improvement. Some of this variation is attributable to genetics and some is due to lifestyle factors (e.g., daily stress level, physical demands of job, eating patterns, alcohol/drug use). Unfortunately there is no way to predict exactly how you will respond to a given training program. It is a process of trial and error. With proper record keeping of all relevant information (workouts, nutrition, supplements, etc.), you will begin to learn which types of training work best for you. It is also important to pay attention to signs of overtraining, like illness, overuse injury, and psychological burn-out. Never ignore what your body is telling you in a misguided effort to stick to a training program at all costs. Make adjustments when necessary.

Reversibility

This is the "use it or lose it" principle. Just as your body can adapt to stress by increasing fitness, it adapts to lack of stress by decreasing it. This effect is referred to as *detraining* by exercise physiologists. The reversibility principle is of particular importance for conditioning as gains in aerobic and anaerobic endurance can rapidly disappear. Research has demonstrated that strength gains from a lifting program can be maintained for several weeks without on-going workouts. However, endurance adaptations can significantly decline after even a few days without training and a return to pre-training levels in only a couple of weeks. This is important information for a couple of reasons. First, it means that no more than a day (possibly two) should be taken off from conditioning work prior to sports performance. Second, after even short vacations you should drop the intensity of the conditioning workouts and ease back into training for the first week or two.

Density

Workout density is defined as the amount of training per unit workout time. The denser a workout, the more you are able to fit into a given block of workout time. Density progression requires you to decrease the time of your rest intervals and move more quickly between sets or exercises. To increase workout density without sacrificing the intensity of each set requires a high work capacity. Gradually increasing the density of your workouts is an excellent way to boost your GPP. You must take time off the rest intervals slowly (follow the 2-week rule) or the average intensity of your sets will drop and compromise their effectiveness. If you can't handle an increase in training quantity without a decrease in quality, then you aren't ready for that volume. Density progression will build your ability to express your strength under conditions of general fatigue, a key factor in sports. It will also allow you to get more training done without staying longer at the gym or adding more training sessions to your schedule.

Training Variables

These variables are used by exercise physiologists and coaches to define and describe training programs. They are widely used in sports science and coaching literature, so it is a good idea to learn what they refer to. Each of these variables must be addressed when creating a program. By manipulating one or more of these variables, you can make slight adjustments to your training or change it entirely.

Mode

Mode refers to the type of exercise performed. Free weights, running, jumping rope, and swimming are all examples of modes. The mode chosen for a given program depends on many different factors:

- *equipment and facilities available* – your resources will determine what options you have in your conditioning program. Look first to improvise with what you have, and then seek to purchase or build equipment that has the greatest versatility

- *specific training goals* – mimic the movements of your sport as closely as possible. For general all-around fitness, rotate many different modes

- *technical knowledge of the athlete* – some modes of exercise require skill in order to perform safely. Never perform an exercise to fatigue without first becoming proficient at it

- *injuries and/or activity restrictions* – chronic or acute illness or injury may contraindicate some exercises for certain people. This is especially true for activities with high impact forces, such as jumping. Be sure to consult a physician before beginning any training and to stop any activity that causes pain

Frequency

Training frequency is how often you work out. Frequency is typically measured in sessions per day and/or sessions per week. Although most trainees will perform only a single daily workout, some particularly hard phases of training might include two or more sessions per day. This is also the case when you combine strength and conditioning sessions with other sports training. Controlling frequency is important to allow enough recovery between sessions and keep total weekly training volume at an optimal level. Noticeable improvements in conditioning are possible with twice-weekly training, so for general fitness 2 to 3 times per week is fine. The more well-trained you are, the higher frequency you can handle.

Intensity

Intensity is a measure of how hard the exercise is relative to your maximal ability for that exercise. For lifts this is typically expressed as a percentage of your 1RM, or the amount of weight that you can lift only once. Endurance intensities are usually expressed as a percentage of VO2 max, or maximal aerobic capacity, with high-intensity work rated above 100%. While the numerical values for intensity matter for research purposes, training intensities can usually be classified for training purposes as maximal, near maximal, moderate, or light efforts for a given repetition range, duration, or distance. Intensity should be increased gradually over time to account for increased fitness. If you use too high an intensity too soon, it may lead to injury or overtraining. It should be noted that intensity is inversely related to both volume and frequency. The harder you work, the less you can do in a given session and the longer you will need to recover between workouts.

Volume

Training volume refers to total workload:

> number of sets * the number of reps * workload per rep

Actual numerical measures of volume are unnecessary unless you are conducting research. For training purposes you can use a more qualitative approach. If you do a lot of reps, sets, or rounds during a training session, it can be considered a high-volume workout and the opposite is true for low volume. What is important to remember is that as volume increases, intensity must go down. You must control the volume in order to maintain intensity throughout the workout. If you are truly giving maximal effort on each rep or bout, then fatigue will accumulate over time. Fatigue progressively reduces your training intensity. Once your training intensity falls below a certain threshold, the session should end. Further work only increases the risk of injury or overtraining and is not training the desired systems anyway. Example thresholds include a cut-off time for sprints or circuits, or the point where the weight cannot be lifted for the desired reps.

Warm-up

You should precede all workouts with a proper warm-up. This statement has often been written but seldom heeded. The goal of the warm-up is to get you physiologically and psychologically ready for training. Skip it and you'll increase your chances of injury and be unable to give a maximal effort. An effective warm-up accomplishes the following goals:

- *increased core and deep muscle temperature* – warm muscle and connective tissue are more pliable, reducing the chances of sprains and strains

- *increased ventilation and heart rate* – heart and lungs get ready to provide all the oxygen and blood you'll need to work out

- *blood shunting* – capillaries feeding the working muscles dilate to bring in more oxygen and fuel and to remove more waste products

- *increased perspiration* – engaging the body's primary cooling mechanism prevents overheating

- *psychological readiness* – when you're warmed-up, you're more motivated to train hard and more likely to recruit more motor units for maximal efforts and have more focus on the activity at hand; plus, you get an endorphin rush and are less likely to notice chronic or nagging pains

To ensure your workouts are as efficient as possible, make sure the warm-up involves useful training. This is a great time to include practice reps of any new movements you are trying to learn. Work any balance training, stability exercises, and prehabilitation or rehabilitation (e.g., neck, rotator cuff, ankles) into the warm-up. Design your warm-up based on the following principles:

1. It accomplishes the physiological goals listed above without undue fatigue.

2. It lasts from 10 to 15 minutes. The more intense the workout, the older the trainee, the earlier in the morning, and the colder the ambient temperature, the longer the warm-up should be.

3. It activates the core muscles and any specific muscle groups that will be trained.

Begin the warm-up by rotating and/or swinging all of your joints through their ranges of motion. Perform 10 to 20 reps of each movement, gradually increasing the range of motion and speed. The following sequence works well and takes about 5 minutes:

Warm-up sequence

- neck – left and right, up and down
- arm swings – cross in front of chest, up and down, single-arm figure eights
- wrist and ankle rotations
- rotator cuff swings – up and down, out to sides
- reaches – touch floor then reach overhead, sidebend, overhead reach
- trunk twists
- hip rotations
- stiff leg swings – front and side
- glute kick
- seated low-back reaches
- hip bridges
- leg chops
- leg across body
- fire hydrants – straight up, circle forward, circle backward
- prone leg-overs

After completing this sequence, all of your joints should be lubricated and ready. Move on to more demanding exercises to get your heart rate and breathing up for the last 5 to 10 minutes. Use a variety of modalities and design the warm-up based on the muscle groups you intend to train. Make sure the load and reps used on any resistance movement are light enough to avoid fatigue. Here are some examples:

Sample warm-up routines

Full-body warm-up circuit (x 3)

jumping jacks	x 15
bodyweight squats	x 10
push-ups	x 10
lat pulldowns	x 10
sit-ups	x 10
back extensions	x 10

Upper-body emphasis warm-up circuit (x 2)

burpees	x 5
DB clean and press	x 10
DB 2-hands swing	x 10
walking lunges	x 10
around the world	x 5/direction
DB deadlift > high pull snatch	x 10
Hindu push-ups	x 5
DB rotating uppercuts	x 10

Lower-body emphasis warm-up circuit (x 2)

step-ups	x 10
good mornings	x 10
DB squat > curl > press	x 5
mountain climbers	x 30
MB Russian twists	x 20
agility ladder runs	3 x 20 ft.
crunches	x 30

In addition to the general warm-up, you should perform one or more warm-up sets for each exercise. As a rule you should do warm-up sets for any exercise in which your work sets have 15 or fewer reps. Start with about 50% of your work weight for at least the same number of reps as your first work set. For lower-intensity work sets, you may only need a single warm-up set, but heavier sets may take four or more.

Sample warm-up sequence for a heavy set of 5

Sets	% of first work set
1 x 10	50%
1 x 8	65%
1 x 5	75%
1 x 5	85%

Cool-down

The cool-down phase of the workout is the opposite of the warm-up. It is designed to bring your heart rate back down to normal and change your mental focus from training back to everyday life. This is also the time to do some static stretching if you need to work on your flexibility. Research shows that static stretching before any activity that requires a high force output may actually make you weaker. Saving it until the end avoids this problem and stretching at this time also typically allows you to stretch farther because your muscles are warm.

A cool-down routine doesn't have to take long: 5 to 10 minutes is sufficient, depending on how much stretching you include. Start with a couple of minutes of walking. Concentrate on your breathing and keep track of your pulse. When your breathing and heart rate come down most of the way, stop and perform some basic joint swings and rotations. Finish with a full-body static stretch. You should perform each static stretch slowly and without bouncing. Go to the point of discomfort (not pain) and hold for 20 to 30 seconds. Do up to 2 to 3 reps if you need to work on your flexibility.

Sample cool-down routine

Walking around and deep breathing

Swings and rotations (x 20 each)
- neck – left and right, up and down
- arm swings – cross in front of chest, up and down, single-arm figure eights
- wrist and ankle rotations
- rotator cuff swings – up and down, out to sides
- reaches – touch floor then reach overhead, side bend, overhead reach
- trunk twists
- hip rotations

Static stretches (hold each stretch for 20–30 sec.)

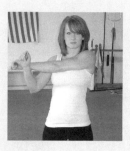

- *shoulder stretch – pull each arm across your chest and hold it with the other arm*

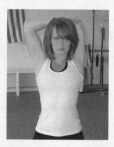

- *triceps stretch – raise your bent arm up beside your head and pull your elbow back with the other arm*

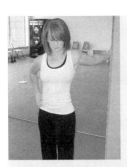

- *pectoral stretch*
  – stand in a door-way and grab both sides with your hands or grab a stationary object with one hand; lean forward and let the weight of your body stretch your chest

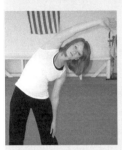

- *sidebend stretch*
  – in a standing position, put one arm over your head and lean to the side; keep your chest forward

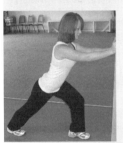

- *calf stretch*
  – stand with one leg forward; keep your back leg straight and your back foot flat on the floor while you press on the wall and bend your front knee

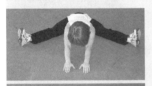
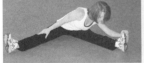

- *seated split stretch* – sit with your legs open wide; stretch by reaching first over the left leg, then the center, then the right leg

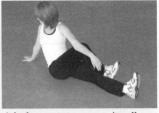

- *spinal twist*
  – sit with one leg straight and the other bent; cross your bent leg over your straight leg; put your opposite elbow on the outside of the bent leg at the knee, and then attempt to turn and look behind you

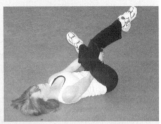

- *piriformis stretch* – lie back with both legs bent; cross the right leg over the left so that the right ankle rests on the left knee; grab behind your left hamstring with both hands and pull the knee towards your head; repeat with the other leg

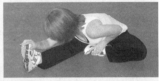

- *modified hurdler stretch* – sit with one leg straight and the other tucked in; lean forward and grab your straight foot or leg

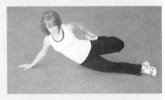

- *quadriceps stretch* – lie on your side; bend your top leg back at the knee, grab your foot, and pull your knee backward

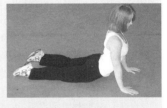

- *cobra stretch* – lie flat on your stomach; put your hands on the floor and push your upper body off the ground; arch your back and look forward or up

Nutrition, Rest, and Restoration

We've already mentioned how important recovery is in the fitness equation. Exercise is a stress which breaks your body down and depletes it. During the period between workouts, your body makes adjustments so that if faced with the same stress again, it is better able to cope. If it isn't given the proper time or materials, your body will not be able to rebuild and replenish itself optimally. You'll go into your next workout beaten down and soon end up in a downward spiral of overtraining and reduced performance. There are three key elements in the recovery recipe: nutrition, rest, and restoration.

Calorie Intake

Raw materials are needed to build anything. If you were going to put an addition on your own house, you'd need to get lumber, nails, and other supplies from a hardware store. If you opted not to get those materials, you would have to tear pieces out of your existing home. Even if you managed to get enough for your addition, the whole house would be weakened and likely to fall apart. Likewise, if you purchased the cheapest building materials for your project, you might compromise the structure's stability. In a very real sense you are what you eat. Improving your fitness is a building project. Protein, fats, and carbohydrates are needed to build bone, muscle, connective tissue, and enzymes, and to restock muscle and liver glycogen stores. If you train hard and don't eat well, you are asking your body to do the impossible—create something out of nothing.

The first part of eating properly is to get enough total calories in your diet. Without them, it doesn't matter what your percentages of protein, fat, and carbohydrates are. Unless you are specifically trying to lose weight, you should eat plenty and eat often. The following equations are quick estimates of resting metabolic rate; they give you the total number of calories your body burns at rest:

men	bodyweight (lb.) x 11
women	bodyweight (lb.) x 10

Using this equation, a 200-lb. man would need 2200 calories. However, this only accounts for resting metabolic rate (RMR). To factor in the calories burned by everyday activity and workouts you can use the following multipliers:

sedentary (little or no activity, desk job)	RMR x 1.2
lightly active (light exercise 1–3 days/week)	RMR x 1.375
moderately active (moderate exercise 3–5 days/week)	RMR x 1.55
very active (hard exercise 6–7 days/week)	RMR x 1.725
extremely active (hard daily exercise)	RMR x 1.9

Let's go back to our 200-lb. man. We will assume he lifts 3 days per week, which would place him in the moderately active category and bump up his calorie requirement to around 3410 per day (2200 x 1.55). If he dropped back on his lifting program he would need less, and if he added in conditioning routines he would need more.

The calorie values provided are estimates and must be adjusted based on how your body responds. If you are attempting to gain or lose weight, then add or subtract 300 to 500 calories from your daily intake. Monitor your weight once a week at the same time immediately after waking up and notice any changes. Make adjustments to your daily intake if necessary.

Macronutrient Profile

Proteins, carbohydrates, and fats are called macronutrients. Eating properly involves taking in enough, but not too much of each of these. Protein is the building material for muscle and many other bodily substances. Without adequate protein, you'll be unable to gain any size and your body will start breaking down your existing muscle to use for enzymes, blood proteins, and the like. Try to get 1 gram of protein for each pound of bodyweight each day. This means that roughly 20 to 25% of your daily calories should come in the form of high-quality protein. The best protein sources include lean meats, chicken, reduced-fat cheeses, milk, and eggs. Animal proteins include all the necessary amino acids. Plant proteins, such as those from soy and legumes, are also acceptable but should not be eaten exclusively. Processed and fried meats should be kept to a minimum, if eaten at all.

Fats are necessary for muscle building and almost all body functions. Unfortunately many people either eat far too much fat, or are so afraid of it that they eat too little. Both of these situations are problematic for health and performance. You should keep your fat intake at around 20 to 30% of your total daily calories. To find what this is in grams, take 30% of your total daily calorie needs and divide it by 9 (fat has 9 calories per gram). Most of the fats you eat should be unsaturated. Unsaturated fats are not associated with heart disease as saturated ones are. In addition, omega-3 fatty acids found in oily fish or flaxseed are heart-protective and may have other health benefits.

Sources of fat

Unsaturated	Saturated
nuts	red meat
seeds	processed meats (bacon, sausage, cold cuts)
flax oil (omega-3)	eggs
salmon (omega-3)	cheese
olives	milk
olive oil	
avocados	

Carbohydrates are the new scapegoat for our unfit, overweight population. The modern popularity of the Atkins and other low-carb diets has demonized carbohydrates in the eyes of many. However, it has gotten a bit out of hand. Very low-carb diets may work well for sedentary people wanting to drop some weight but not for those who are extremely active. The fact is, if you plan to be a well-conditioned athlete, you must eat some carbs to fuel your training. Currently there are many hotly debated recommendations about carbohydrate intake; this book takes a middle road. I suggest the following guidelines:

1. Avoid refined sugar. Sugars such as high-fructose corn syrup have an almost drug-like effect on your insulin levels, turning you into a fat storage machine. Eating refined sugar also causes major fluctuations in your energy level, with brief "highs" followed by fatigue, irritability, and hunger. Eliminate as much refined sugar from your diet as possible. There are two exceptions to this general rule. First, a sugared sports beverage may be consumed during or immediately after your workout. At this time, the sugar will not affect your hormone levels as much. Second, you can opt to establish one cheat meal per week if you must have a sugar fix.

2. Eat whole fruit rather than drinking juice. Fruit juice is a very concentrated form of sugar that has an effect on fat storage and energy levels similar to refined sugar. Whole fruit contains fiber which helps stabilize blood sugar.

3. Eat mostly whole grain, unprocessed carbohydrates. Breads and pastas made with processed white flour have an effect on your hormones similar to sugar. Trade them in for whole grain products.

4. Try to eat a balance of macronutrients at each meal. Meals based around carbohydrates (such as pizza, pasta, or some sort of light sauce served over rice) usually do not have enough protein. Carb-based meals are also often lacking in vitamins and minerals.

5. Eat more green, fibrous or leafy vegetables. Veggies such as broccoli, cauliflower, asparagus, and green beans have a lot of fiber and vitamins. Try to include a few servings at each meal.

Micronutrients

Micronutrients are vitamins, minerals, and other substances required by the body for normal functioning. In a perfect world we should get most of what we need from whole foods. However, few people eat enough variety to ensure this. Factor in that cooking and processing remove many nutrients, and it is easy to come up short. The remedy is simple: buy a high-quality multi-vitamin and take it daily. This way if you miss something in your diet, you'll be sure to get it. Aside from these, there may be reasons to get more of a few other nutrients.

The following vitamins and minerals have either been shown to be depleted by physical exercise or needed in higher quantities by those who exercise frequently:

	Take daily
Vitamin C	500 mg – 1000 mg
Vitamin E	400 IU
Zinc	25 mg

Vitamin C and E boost immune function and act as antioxidants that protect you against the free radical molecules produced during training. There is also some evidence that C and E can help protect against delayed-onset muscle soreness. Athletes can benefit from taking these at higher than the recommended daily allowance (RDA) for the average sedentary individual.

Hydration

Your body is about 70% water. Water is lost throughout the day through breathing, sweating, and the elimination of waste products. When you exercise, particularly in a hot and/or humid environment, sweat rate rises dramatically. If you don't actively replace the lost water, you'll become dehydrated and your health and performance will suffer. Drink at least one glass of plain water with each meal and drink water before, during, and after your workouts. Alcoholic beverages and other drugs like caffeine act as diuretics, so you may have to drink more water to compensate.

Relying on your thirst is not the best way to stay hydrated. The thirst mechanism is a negative feedback loop, meaning you won't get thirsty until you are already somewhat dehydrated. Try to prevent this by drinking water throughout the day. Other than thirst, the easiest way to tell your hydration status is by the frequency and color of your urine. If you go frequently throughout the day and it is lightly colored or clear, you're fine. However, if it is infrequent or dark yellow, you most likely need more water.

Workout Formats

Within the context of the basic training principles already presented, there are many ways to implement a conditioning program. Conditioning work can be kept separate from strength and power training, done back to back, or integrated with heavy lifting. There is no best way for all situations and trainees. All of these methods are effective, but some will fit your particular circumstances better than others. Additionally, it is important to rotate the workout format regularly so that your training stays fresh and interesting. Many will scoff at the idea that workouts should be "interesting," asserting that everyone should just plow through the basic exercises and deal with it. However, if your workouts become boring and tedious, you will find it difficult to put much into them and the likelihood of your skipping training sessions increases. There are far too many ways to train for you to stick to the same plan all the time.

Designing workouts is about balancing the opposing forces of consistency and variety. *Consistency* in training means that there is an overall training goal and that all of the workouts move you toward that goal. Without it, your training will disintegrate into series of pointless, random training sessions. *Variety* is the intentional rotation of training methods and formats. This is ideal for preventing physical and mental burnout as well as helping to avoid overuse injuries and muscle imbalances.

Circuit Training

The first formalized system of circuit training was developed by Morgan and Adamson, two British physical educators, and was published in their 1957 book *Circuit Training*. Their circuit program used an assortment of free weight, bodyweight, and gymnastics exercises sequenced to build strength and endurance simultaneously. Unfortunately circuit training today is often synonymous with low-intensity, high-rep toning routines performed exclusively on weight machines. The pec deck chest machine has replaced bodyweight dips and seated machine rows have supplanted rope climbing, dramatically reducing modern circuit training's effectiveness and functionality.

Circuit training is actually a very efficient and versatile method of combining conditioning work with strength and/or muscular hypertrophy training. *All that is absolutely required for circuit training is that you perform the exercises in a sequence.* You complete a single set of each exercise in order before starting over at the beginning, rather than performing all sets of an exercise before moving to the next one. A circuit consists of at least three different exercises. Circuits with only two exercises are traditionally called supersets.

The physiological rationale behind circuit training is to minimize specific fatigue while accumulating general fatigue. Specific fatigue refers to fatigue of the exercised muscle groups. If you were bench pressing, specific fatigue would be that of the triceps, shoulders, pectorals, and other involved muscle groups. The exact cause of the fatigue will depend on the loads and rep ranges used, with higher-rep fatigue resulting from the accumulation of lactic acid and lower-rep fatigue more from neural factors.

General fatigue is typically fatigue of the cardio-respiratory system and whole-body blood lactate levels. It is associated with increased heart rate, breathing rate, and sweating. The exercised muscle groups are typically rotated during a circuit so that there is a local recovery or decrease in specific fatigue, with increases over time in general fatigue due to continuous activity. Heart rate and breathing remain elevated throughout the training session, resulting in increased aerobic and anaerobic endurance.

Here are some factors to consider when designing circuits:

1. *Goals of the training program* – though a complete discussion of strength training programming is beyond the scope of this book, suffice it to say that the exercises, loads, and repetition ranges you choose should be consonant with your training goals.

2. *Circuit flow and facility layout* – with circuit training perhaps more than any other type of workout, it is important to keep in mind the physical layout of your gym. Make sure that exercises that follow one another in the workout use equipment or spaces that are in close proximity. Because rest between exercises and sets is a major factor in circuits, having to walk all the way across the room might allow too much rest. If you are designing a circuit to be used by a group of athletes, be sure it follows an obvious path and the stations are clearly marked; otherwise, what looked so good on paper will fall apart in practice.

3. *Crowd control* – if you train in a crowded commercial gym, you'll have to factor that in to any program design. Once you get off a piece of equipment, there'll be no guarantee that it will be unoccupied when you need it again. If your gym is crowded, you have fewer options. First, consider using some other training format besides the circuit. Alternatively, you can break what would be a larger circuit into a series of supersets or mini-circuits. You could also write a program that utilizes portable equipment (such as dumbbells, medicine balls, and jump ropes) that you could feasibly cart off to a remote corner of the gym until you're finished.

4. *Flexibility* – the key to a successful circuit workout is to keep moving. Occasionally in a commercial gym, interruptions will occur. Someone may be using the equipment you need when you get there or hop on it when you take a water break. If this happens, immediately go to a plan B exercise. Use a lift that is similar to the one you were supposed to do. For instance, instead of pull-ups do lat pulldowns, upright rows, or bent-over rows. Don't get upset or try to discuss the situation with the other person; just go seamlessly into your alternate lift.

Creating circuit workouts

Circuit training lends itself well to all types of exercise modalities. You can easily incorporate weight machines, free weights, calisthenics, jumping rope, running, and anything else into a circuit. Any combination of these modalities can be mixed together as well. The many different ways to approach circuit training will depend on your preferences and goals:

1. *Number of exercises* – with a given volume of training you can either go through a smaller circuit more times or a longer circuit fewer times. A 3-exercise mini-circuit could be done 5 or more times in a workout while you may only need to go through a 15-exercise circuit once. Use fewer exercises to provide maximal overload on a smaller set of muscle fibers and more exercises to train a larger amount of muscle mass.

2. *Rest intervals* – vary the rest between exercises in the circuit or trips through the circuit. For maximal conditioning benefit, use as little rest as possible while still maintaining the required intensity and getting all the reps in each set.

3. *Mixed modes* – traditional circuit programs use a series of lifts, but you can also incorporate other types of exercises. For instance, follow dumbbell overhead pressing with a 400-meter sprint, 60 seconds of jumping rope, or a set of cartwheels.

4. *Alternating intensity* – within a circuit, all the exercises do not have to be equally difficult. The more muscle mass or movement involved in an exercise, the greater the fatigue it will induce. Compare the effect of a set of 10 biceps curls on your heart rate with the effect produced by a set of 10 power cleans. You can take advantage of this to scale the intensity of your workouts. Alternate more and less intense exercises to provide some recovery. Bump up the intensity by placing demanding exercises next to one another.

The following section contains some different circuit designs and applications to help you come up with your own programs.

The original circuit training program

This is the original circuit training program described in Morgan and Adamson's 1957 book, *Circuit Training*. The workouts below are taken from this book and represent four different variations. Although most of the exercises are standard, a few are described in the book and may need some clarification:

- stepping – step-ups onto a box or bench
- jump and heave – using the legs to assist in jumping into the top position of the chin-up
- jump and press – using the legs to jump into an arm lock-out position on high dip or parallel bars
- rope swings – swinging back and forth by holding onto two climbing ropes, one in each hand
- dumbbell raising sideways – dumbbell lateral raise for the shoulders
- wheelbarrow lift – a deadlifting device depicted in the book; it can be simulated by deadlifts or partial deadlifts with a trap bar (parallel grip)

Circuit intensity and workload can be adjusted by changing dumbbell or barbell weight, number of repetitions, or number of trips through the circuit, or by completing the circuit in a certain time.

Circuit Variations (Morgan & Adamson)

Normal
1. stepping
2. burpee
3. jump and heave
4. trunk curls
5. dumbbell jumps
6. barbell curls
7. dumbbell squats
8. jump and press
9. rope swings

Tough
1. stepping
2. squat thrusts
3. chinning
4. trunk curls
5. wheelbarrow lift (parallel-grip deadlift)
6. wrist rolling
7. barbell squats
8. dips
9. rope swings

Short
1. stepping
2. jump and heave
3. trunk curls
4. barbell curls
5. jump and press
6. rope swings

Long
1. stepping
2. squat thrusts
3. chinning
4. trunk curls
5. dumbbell raising sideways
6. squat jumps
7. wheelbarrow lift (parallel-grip deadlift)
8. wrist rolling
9. dumbbell squats
10. barbell press
11. rope swings
12. rope ladder climb

Strength training circuits

The most effective way to build strength is by lifting heavy weights for low repetitions using large, multi-joint free-weight exercises. Although there is no established "best" repetition range for strength work, you should generally keep the repetitions to 8 or fewer and utilize loads between 80 to 100% of your max. The best exercises for limit strength training are those that use the maximum amount of muscle mass, such as squats, deadlifts, cleans, snatches, bent rows, pull-ups, bench presses, overhead presses, and dips. The typical strength program calls for up to 3 to 5 minutes of rest between heavy sets of the same exercise.

For the strength circuit, you adhere to this guideline as well. However, instead of complete, passive recovery, you perform exercises for other body parts during this time. The key is to choose additional exercises that will allow you to rest the muscles used in the heavy set. It is okay for the other exercises to involve the resting muscles to some degree, just not so much that you cannot recover properly. It is important to remember that general fatigue will interfere with specific strength. If you are new to circuit work or conditioning and your GPP levels are low, you will likely notice a drop in your training weights. This may be a blow to your ego, but it is normal. As you get in better shape, you will be able to express your specific strength under conditions of general fatigue, and the weights will climb back up to where they were. Take a look at the following pressing workout:

Specific strength circuit focusing on pressing

- military press x 5
- BB biceps curls x 12
- jumping jacks x 30
- incline sit-ups x 15
- back extensions x 15
- bodyweight squats x 25

In this workout, a heavy set of military presses is followed by five additional exercises for the rest of the body performed at higher reps. Of the five, biceps curls involve the greatest muscle group overlap and thus are placed immediately after the pressing. This allows maximum arm and shoulder recovery before the next heavy set. The above workout would be performed in circuit fashion 3 to 5 times through with no (or minimal) rest between circuits. Remember to warm up properly for any low-rep, high-intensity strength circuit. Use a standard warm-up set progression for your heavy lift before beginning the circuit. Warm-up sets for the lighter, higher-rep exercises are unnecessary.

More than one heavy exercise can be performed in a given workout if the circuit is set up correctly. The next circuit includes heavy lifts for all major muscle groups. Keep in mind that there will be some fatigue interference when setting up a workout such as this, but the efficiency and conditioning benefits more than make up for slightly diminished training weights. Again, after warming up for the heavy lifts, you would perform this circuit up to 5 times with little or no rest between circuits.

Circuit with heavy lifts for all muscle groups

- weighted pull-ups x 3
- Russian twists x 20
- back squats x 1
- jump rope x 50 hits
- flat BB bench press x 3
- reverse hypers x 15
- burpees x 8

Hypertrophy training circuits

If your primary training goal is an increase in muscle mass, your circuit design must be modified. Hypertrophy training can be thought of as *volume* overload as opposed to *intensity* overload. In other words, workouts should be designed to cause the maximum amount of local muscular fatigue to a particular body part or muscle group to force it to grow. This is accomplished by working the trained areas to the limits of their capacity and sometimes slightly beyond, so that as many muscle fibers are recruited as possible. Hypertrophy work requires a slightly higher repetition range, lower loads, and often more than a single exercise for a given muscle group. As in strength training, multi-joint exercises should form the foundation of the workout, but isolation training is useful to ensure all areas are overloaded maximally. Due to the higher volume demands per muscle group, it is useful to do some sort of training split. The following is an example of a hypertrophy workout emphasizing the lower body:

Lower body volume overload circuit

- BB back squat   x 10
- weighted crunch   x 25
- glute ham raise   x 12
- DB biceps curl to overhead press   x 15
- leg extension   x 12
- back extension   x 15
- seated calf raise   x 15

Advanced hypertrophy techniques

Various hypertrophy techniques can easily be incorporated into the circuit training workout. As with any training program, you must pay attention to your total workout volume and use these intensification methods judiciously to avoid overtraining. It is not recommended that you train to failure on every workout.

• **Supersets or stacking** – This is placing two or more exercises for the same muscle group in a series with no rest between. The actual movements are different but hit mostly the same fibers to thoroughly exhaust that muscle. The following workout for chest, triceps, and shoulders demonstrates how multiple exercises for the same body part can be stacked to provide more overload:

Chest, triceps, and shoulders workout

- BB flat bench press   x 12
- DB incline bench press   x 12
- DB overhead press   x 12
- DB fly   x 12
- triceps pressdown (rope)   x 12
- DB side delt raise   x 12

• **Drop sets** – As you complete a set of moderate to high repetitions (8 reps or more), your muscles fatigue. This is the reason that the final reps in the set are much more difficult. By stripping off some of the weight at the end of the set you can continue, squeezing out even more repetitions. This is the principle behind the drop set. Once you hit failure, have your training partner quickly strip off 10 to 20% of the load and continue until you hit failure again. Repeat this process one or more times to thoroughly exhaust the muscles. If you are alone, you can quickly switch the pin on a weight stack or grab a lighter set of dumbbells. Rest those muscles as you complete the intervening exercises. Here is an example of an upper-body pulling workout using this technique. A repetition range is given only for the first set because for each subsequent set, you try to complete as many reps as possible:

Upper-body pulling workout

• BB bent-over row drop set	x 10–12 (3 drops)
• jumping jack	x 30
• bodyweight squat	x 25
• DB shrug	x 15
• incline sit-up	x 15

• **Forced repetitions** – These are based on a principle similar to the drop set. When you reach failure on an exercise, your spotter provides just enough assistance to allow you to get several more repetitions, usually 4 to 8. Tell your lifting partner beforehand how many additional reps you plan to do so he will know when you are finished.

• **Cheat repetitions** – Another set extender method to compensate for fatigue, cheat reps involve changing the technique of the lift when you hit failure to enable you to keep going. "Cheating" on a repetition does not mean moving the weight however you can. The cheat is actually a new version of the lift and must be done with proper technique to avoid injury. The first method of cheating is by using leg drive or hip explosion. Thus an overhead press becomes a push press or jerk, or an upright row becomes a high pull. The second method is by shortening the range of motion. Rather than bringing the dumbbells all the way down in the bench press, start doing one-half presses or go from full squats to one-quarter squats. Once you hit technical failure on the cheat version, end the set.

Peripheral heart action

Peripheral heart action (PHA) training is a type of circuit training developed in the 1960s as a method for bodybuilders to drop body fat while maintaining muscle mass. With PHA you do circuits of basic lifts for high repetitions sequenced so that you rotate body parts on each lift. This builds a high level of general fatigue while allowing for local muscular recovery. The premise of PHA workouts is to keep the blood continually moving throughout the body. In a typical high-volume hypertrophy program, several sets or exercises are performed in a row for a single muscle group. This causes an intense "pump" as blood is rerouted to the area. The pump may last for a long time after the workout is over, evidence of blood pooling in those muscles. When muscle becomes active, the capillary beds dilate and blood flow to the area increases. PHA takes advantage of this by rotating muscle groups during lifting to send blood from one end of the body to the other. Ideally the muscle groups are rotated so that those that follow one another are as far apart as possible.

PHA training serves its intended purpose well. It can strip off body fat in record time and let you hold on to your hard-earned muscle mass. However, that is not the end of its usefulness. PHA makes a great muscular endurance and general conditioning training protocol. It also allows you to take a break from heavy lifting for a few weeks. You can incorporate a week or two of PHA or other circuit training after every 6 to 8 weeks of high-load training.

PHA works best with sets of 10 or more reps and lifts that emphasize only one main area of the body. The idea is for you to maximize the blood flow to a given muscle group during the set. Lower repetitions do not induce the same amount of blood flow to an area as higher repetitions do. Compound lifts or those that hit muscle groups throughout the body are very tiring but do not direct the blood anywhere in particular. Avoid using lifts such as the clean and jerk, squat press, or Turkish get-up. Instead opt for overhead presses, squats, pull-ups, and other more localized movements.

The weight you use during PHA training should be challenging, but do not train to failure on any set. Scale the difficulty of the PHA workouts by increasing or decreasing: 1) reps per set; 2) number of exercises per circuit; 3) number of trips through the circuit; and 4) resistance on each exercise.

The following is one example of a PHA workout. Do this workout 3 to 5 times through with minimal, if any, rest between exercises and circuits. Notice the rotation of exercises from upper to lower body:

PHA circuit

- BB squat   x 15
- DB bench press   x 15
- incline sit-up   x 20
- lat pulldown   x 15
- leg curl   x 15
- DB overhead press   x 15
- back extension   x 20
- seated cable row   x 15
- leg extension   x 15
- DB triceps extension   x 15
- DB side bend   x 15/side
- BB curl   x 15

20-Rep Sets

In his book *SUPER SQUATS: How to Gain 30 Pounds of Muscle in 6 Weeks*, Randall Strossen outlines one of the most effective hypertrophy programs ever created. For all its effectiveness, this routine is exceptionally simple. It is based around a single set or two of heavy barbell squats done for 20 consecutive repetitions. You load up a bar with a weight you would normally use for a set of 10, and then grind out 20 reps before you rack it. As the reps climb, you pause for a few seconds after each one and take some deep breaths before moving on. On each consecutive workout you strive to add weight to the bar. There is more to the program than this, but the squats are really the *pièce de résistance*.

In addition to muscle mass, 20-rep squatting has a tremendous conditioning effect on your entire body. As the weight climbs, the sets can take 5 minutes or more to complete. This increase not only builds leg endurance, but also overloads the phosphagen and glycolytic systems maximally. After a few weeks of these sets, your lactic acid tolerance and anaerobic endurance will improve dramatically.

Back squats are not the only lifts that can be trained using the 20-rep system. Admittedly having to keep the bar on your back between reps makes back squats particularly brutal, but any lift that involves a lot of muscle mass and allows a reasonable load will work. Some suggested lifts are:

- heavy quarter squats
- front squats
- Hack squats
- deadlifts
- trap bar deadlifts
- clean pulls from floor
- snatch pulls from floor
- Turkish get-ups

For an extended workout using the 20-rep principle, use complex lifts that include multiple movements for all of the major muscle groups. For the following it is recommended that you take several seconds of rest between each rep. The goal of the workout is to complete all 20 reps in the shortest time possible.

- clean and jerk
- power clean – front squat – push press
- power snatch – back squat – jerk from behind neck

Pay close attention to your form when doing any high-rep sets with any of these lifts. Failure occurs when you can no longer complete reps with decent form. Pushing beyond this point puts you at great risk of injury, particularly in your shoulders and lower back.

Interval Training

Interval training involves alternating periods of work (work intervals) with periods of recovery (rest intervals). The basic idea behind it is that by including rest intervals, more total high-intensity work can be accomplished during a workout than if no recovery were allowed. During typical low-intensity endurance work such as jogging, mostly slow-twitch muscle fibers are used and fast-twitch fibers receive very little training. The increased intensity of interval workouts allows you to condition the fast-twitch fibers.

Interval training has been traditionally used by endurance athletes to improve speed and anaerobic capacity for the final all-out "kick" at the end of a race; or by athletes, such as football players and wrestlers, whose sports require short, intense effort followed by periods of inactivity or low-intensity effort. Interval training builds your capacity for intense work both physiologically and psychologically. Physiologically you will produce less lactic acid at a given work intensity and have greater capacity to buffer it; and psychologically you will be better able to tolerate the painful, adverse effects of high blood lactic acid.

Recent research has also demonstrated high-intensity interval training to be as effective as long duration, moderate-intensity aerobic work for increasing aerobic capacity and may be more effective for losing body fat. Interval workouts also typically take much less time than long, slow, distance work, making them ideal for anyone with limited training time.

Interval duration

Generally speaking, there is a direct relationship between the intensity of the work interval and the duration of the rest interval. In other words, if you work harder, you will need to rest longer. The table below gives some suggested guidelines for work to rest intervals based on interval intensity. It is important to remember that interval workouts should not allow for complete recovery but just enough for you to complete the next maximal effort. As you accumulate more reps in a workout, you will get more and more fatigued and have a tendency to want to rest more. If you do not have a coach or workout partner to push you, invest in a timer or clock to keep your intervals consistent.

Work to rest intervals based on intensity

Intensity	Work time	Work to rest ratios
maximal	5–10 sec.	1:10–1:15
high	15–30 sec.	1:3–1:5
medium	60–120 sec.	1:3–1:5
low	> 120 sec.	1:1–1:2

Passive vs. active recovery

Rest intervals can involve either passive or active recovery. Passive recovery is complete rest: you just sit or stand there until you are ready to go again. Active recovery involves performing low-intensity work during the rest interval. We know that the point of passive recovery is to rest completely and conserve energy before the next bout. What is the point of active recovery?

Active recovery serves a twofold purpose. First, it adds additional aerobic training without increasing the length of the workout. More training means more improvement. Second, it actually helps speed up recovery. One of the primary causes of fatigue during short, high-intensity exercise is the accumulation of lactic acid. In addition to the subjective feelings of pain, burning, and nausea it can produce, the lowered blood pH can interfere with muscle contraction. However, lactic acid is not entirely bad. It can be taken up and used for fuel by oxidative (slow twitch) or heart muscle fibers, or reconverted to glucose in the liver. Light activity speeds up these processes and, thus, lactic acid levels are reduced much faster.

For maximum effectiveness, use of active recovery in interval workouts must be governed by three basic guidelines:

1. *Fitness level* – Even with a reduced intensity, additional work may be too much if you don't have a sufficient conditioning base. Until you have a few weeks of training, do not do anything more than walk around slowly.

2. *Relative intensity* – Make sure that the recovery activity does not cause additional fatigue. As a general rule, the higher the work intensity, the lower the recovery intensity.

3. *Exercise mode* – Choose a recovery mode that allows a quick transition from work to active recovery. Intervals are typically measured in seconds so you should not waste time fumbling around with new equipment or relocating to the other side of the gym.

Progression

As with any type of physical training, you must build up your interval training volume and intensity gradually to prevent overtraining and/or injury. Start with moderate-intensity work intervals and gradually build up by (a) increasing work interval intensity, (b) decreasing the rest interval, or (c) increasing the number of work intervals per workout. A good rule of thumb is to progress slightly for every 2 weeks of consistent training. Consistent means that you actually complete all of the workouts you have planned. If you miss one or more workouts in a given 2-week period, do not increase the intensity. Never allow what you have planned on paper to get in the way of reality. After any complete layoff of 2 weeks or more, decrease the intensity and build back up. How much you need to drop back will depend on how long a break you took. Use a build-up period at least equal to the time of your layoff. This guideline is especially important with regard to conditioning. You do not lose strength nearly as fast as endurance. Endurance can begin dropping significantly in as little time as a week.

Exercise mode

Interval training works well with a variety of different modes. Your choice of exercises will depend on your available equipment and particular training goals. Always remember that the principle of specificity applies to conditioning training. Any exercise that gets your heart and breathing rate up will promote cardiovascular adaptation; muscles that are not used in the training activity will receive little benefit. If your goal is sport-specific conditioning, you should emphasize movements and exercises most like those you must do in competition. If you are not training for a specific sport but rather for all-around conditioning or fat loss, including a wide variety of different exercises is ideal. Exercise modes can be mixed within workouts, between workouts, or from week to week. Here are some examples of suitable exercises:

Exercise modes for general fitness

- running
- swimming
- rowing
- Versa-Climber
- cycling
- heavy bag rounds
- calisthenics
- free weight lifts

Tabata intervals

A 1996 study by Japanese researcher Izumi Tabata and his colleagues found that 20 seconds of maximal exercise followed by 10 seconds of active recovery repeated 6 to 8 times produced cardiovascular improvements comparable to much more time-consuming moderate-intensity aerobic training protocols. Thus was born the Tabata interval. Although the original study used resisted cycling, this name has been applied to any interval program based on the 20-second work and 10-second rest schedule.

The short duration of this protocol requires all-out effort during the work intervals. For this reason it is recommended that you first build up a base with lower-intensity training before beginning a program this intense. The subjects in the original study were recreationally-trained physical education students, suggesting that 6 to 8 repetitions performed 2 to 3 times weekly is a good place to start. Following the principle of slow, steady progression discussed earlier, add a repetition or two every couple of weeks.

Exercises that involve a lot of muscle mass are the best choices for Tabata intervals. Running, cycling, or rowing sprints; dumbbell or barbell squats; thrusters or deadlifts; or bodyweight calisthenics such as burpees work well. Whatever your mode, you must be able to make the transition from work to rest very quickly because the intervals are so short. You must also be able to clearly see or hear your interval timer or clock. If possible, have a training partner keep time for you during these workouts.

Fartlek running

Fartlek is a Swedish term that means "speed play." It was popularized as a training method for distance runners in the 1930s. *Fartlek* is a type of intuitive interval training. Rather than set-ting up a rigid schedule of work and rest intervals for the workout, you go on a run of 15 minutes or more and mix up slow running, moderate running, and sprinting at random. If you run outdoors, you can use environmental objects like trees or lampposts to mark distances. Incorporate hill or stair runs, jog backwards, or stop briefly and throw in some shadowboxing like Rocky Balboa. This method works well for more advanced athletes who are willing and able to work hard. The major drawback to *fartlek* training is that it is easy to slack off when you fatigue.

Fartlek training can be done with exercises other than running. Rowing, cycling, swimming, or various cardio machines can be used. Many of these come with a built-in "random" interval training workout for which the computer generates an interval workout on the spot that is different each time. These programs are based on the *fartlek* concept.

Interval timers

Interval training is based on pre-selected segments of time, which means that you will need some way to tell when to start and stop. There are a number of ways you can do this.

1. *Interval timer* – You can purchase many different interval timers through sports supply companies. The top-end ones have large numerical LED displays and can be programmed to count off any duration interval you want. The drawback to these is the expense. You can find less expensive timers from boxing supply companies. These usually have settings for 2- to 3-minute rounds and 30-second to 1-minute rests. They typically cannot be programmed but are much less expensive. They can be used in combination with a clock with a second hand to time shorter intervals within a round.

2. *Cooking timers* – These are small, programmable electronic timers for kitchen use. Although they vary in the features offered, most can be used to count up or down to any time up to 99 minutes and 59 seconds, alerting you with a beep when finished. Cooking timers are very portable and inexpensive.

3. *Clock* – A clock with a visible second hand is a great way to time short intervals such as Tabatas. Put the clock in a position where you can see it during all of your exercises. The only drawbacks are that it won't have a bell to alert you when the round is over and it can be easy to lose track of the time on longer rounds.

4. *Personalized CD* – Make a CD of your favorite songs that plays for a certain time and then has a period of silence to indicate rest intervals. Alternatively, you could choose songs of particular lengths to represent rounds.

5. *Coach or training partner* – If possible, have a coach or training partner time you with a stopwatch. Next to a programmable interval timer, this is the best option because you only have to worry about training, not keeping track of the time.

Finishers

Finishers are exercises done at the end of a normal workout to use up your last remaining bit of energy. They are usually a single set done to complete failure. Finishers are extremely beneficial if performed sparingly, but using them too often can easily lead to overtraining. The physiological benefits are, first, that the extreme fatigue forces your body to recruit all motor units, even the high-threshold reserves. Second, finishers train more than just the body, they also train your mind. Psychologically, finishers teach you to push through your limits. They are self-imposed tests of mental toughness that will help you overcome training plateaus. Third, the finisher, like 1RM testing, serves to chart your strength–endurance or anaerobic progress.

Design specific finisher workouts to be completed every few months. During these, your goal is to give it everything you have in an effort to beat your old score and set a new PR. Finishers are repetition or duration efforts performed with a challenging but sub-maximal load. Most use a full-body exercise but it is also possible to do a finisher with a specific lift done earlier in the workout. Some examples include:

- max reps on bench press, deadlift, squat, etc.
- max reps on kettlebell/dumbbell cleans, snatches, or push presses
- timed mile run
- max 100 m sprints in a given time
- bodyweight lunge walk for max distance or reps
- heavy sandbag shouldering or cleaning for max reps
- heavy sandbag carries for maximal time or distance
- heavy sandbag loading onto a platform for max reps
- dragging sled or sandbag for max distance
- tire flip for max reps or distance
- max consecutive burpee reps without resting or max reps in a given time

If you have a training partner who is at about the same fitness level as you, then competitive finishers will help give you additional motivation. Compete against each other for time, distance, reps, or duration. Carries, drags, sandbag lifts, tire flips, and repeated sprint races all lend themselves to this type of workout. You can also use the "I go, you go" format and take turns with an exercise until one of you doesn't make his set. This competitive element can really bump up the intensity of your workout. If one person is in much better shape, then he can pace the workout, forcing the other to push harder.

Keep the following guidelines in mind when using finishers:

- Use finishers only occasionally – Because finishers require so much physical and mental effort, it is easy to overtrain if you do them too frequently. They also usually cause a great deal of soreness and that can interfere with other workouts. One finisher set every couple of weeks is plenty.

- Pay attention to technique – Only use exercises that you can perform with excellent technique. If fatigue begins to interfere too severely with your form, then consider that failure. It is better to forego the last few reps than to take the chance of injuring yourself.

Training Groups or Teams

If you are a coach or instructor, you'll often need to design workouts for an entire team or class. This can be challenging, especially if your equipment is limited or not everyone is at the same fitness level. It is not an impossible task though as long as you think it out ahead of time. Let's consider some of the problems that can arise and possible solutions for dealing with them.

Limited equipment

Most coaches will face this problem at some point or other in their careers. In an ideal world this wouldn't be a problem: you would have everything you needed all the time to implement your ideas. However, in reality funding and facilities are often scarce. Either you have a poorly equipped gym, no gym, or far too many athletes for the resources you have available. Here are ways to make the best of this situation:

1. If you have any money available for equipment, the following items are relatively inexpensive and make for great group training. One of the greatest benefits is that they are portable: you can move your gym anywhere you need it.

- Dumbbells – buy these used at garage sales or sporting consignment stores. Try to get as many pairs between 15 lb. and 35 lb. as you can. Most of the exercises for conditioning work will use these weights
- Sandbags – make several sandbags of different weights from 50 lb. all the way to 150 lb. If you can, make one sandbag of each weight for every two athletes
- Jump ropes – these are inexpensive enough for you to require every athlete to buy one for his/her own use
- Orange marker cones – use them for setting up circuits, running, or agility drills
- Rubber bands and tubing – if possible, get at least one for every pair of athletes

2. Conduct conditioning sessions in a nearby park, preferably one with hills or playground equipment.

3. Learn and use as many bodyweight and partner resistance exercises as possible.

4. Form pairs or trios of athletes around a single piece of equipment. One uses the equipment while the others rest or use bodyweight exercises. Keep track of time rather than reps and have them switch places on your signal.

Supervision

Keeping track of what all the athletes are doing is essential for preventing injury and keeping them from slacking off. Consider this when you set up your conditioning area. For in-place repetition work, have the athletes form a semi-circle with you in front. From this viewpoint you will be able to see everyone at once. Use a stopwatch to time intervals and for repetitions, have the athletes keep the same pace: count the repetitions and have everyone count back.

For moving circuits or other drills, position yourself centrally so that you can take in the whole scene with minimal effort. Get an assistant coach if possible, or make use of the older or more motivated athletes to push the others.

Differing fitness levels

Consider breaking your team into two different groups based on fitness. The ideal situation is to create separate workouts appropriate for each group and train them during different sessions. If this is not feasible, write a workout using as many exercises as possible that work for both groups, selecting exercises that can be easily modified by changing the load, repetitions, rest intervals, or intensities. Dumbbells, kettlebells, resistance bands, sandbags, and body-weight exercises all work well.

Regulating Workout Effort

Both objective and subjective methods exist for regulating workout intensity. Many people choose to regulate their workout intensity subjectively. If the session calls for a one-mile run, you could run it as fast as possible or at a more moderate pace. The first intensity would represent 100% while the second a somewhat lower percentage, depending on how much you put into it. This is the easiest way to determine your intensity but also the least accurate. If you are an advanced trainee, you will be able to use this system much more effectively than if you are a novice.

Rating of Perceived Exertion (RPE)

A more accurate subjective rating system commonly used in exercise physiology is the Rating of Perceived Exertion Scale. Designed by researcher Gunnar Borg, this scale has been validated in numerous studies. This numerical scale has a direct and linear relationship to intensity measured as a percentage of one's maximal aerobic output. Each number represents a level of effort as perceived by the trainee. The revised version of Borg's scale runs from 0 to 10, with 0 representing rest and maximum effort being above 10.

Borg's Rating of Perceived Exertion Scale

0	Nothing at all
0.5	Very, very light (just noticeable)
1	Very light
2	Light (weak)
3	Moderate
4	Somewhat hard
5	Heavy (strong)
6	
7	Very heavy
8	
9	
10	Very, very heavy (almost max)
	Maximal

Using this scale, intensity can be divided into four main zones:

1. *Warm-up zone (RPE 1–3)* – You should be here after a proper warm-up and never dip below this during a workout. If you do, it means you have cooled off too much. This zone is too low for any significant fitness improvements.

2. *Low zone (RPE 3–6)* – Training in this zone works primarily aerobic energy systems. There will be little net lactic acid accumulation. If you are doing continuous bouts of exercise for 15 minutes or more, this zone is appropriate.

3. *Medium zone (RPE 6–8)* – At this level, the emphasis shifts from aerobic to anaerobic energy systems. Lactic acid accumulates and fatigue can become severe.

4. *High zone (RPE 8–max)* – This zone represents an all-out effort. Your body's anaerobic energy production and lactic acid tolerance will be stressed maximally. This pace can only be continued for very short intervals.

After a few sessions, you'll be able to calibrate the scale effectively. For the first few weeks, learn to associate values on the RPE with different workouts, making notes of this in your training journal. Very soon you'll be able to specify RPE values (or intensity zones) beforehand and have no trouble staying at the proper intensity. If you are coaching a group of athletes, make a large RPE wall chart that everyone can see during the training session. Calibrate it for a couple of weeks by pushing your athletes to specific intensities and then pointing out at which level they are on the chart. After a while, you'll be able to give them a numerical value (or zone) and have them match it consistently.

Heart rate

Some people prefer a more objective measure of exercise intensity than perceived or maximal effort. Heart rate provides a ready method of quantifying intensity. There is a direct relationship between how hard you work and how high your heart rate goes. Working muscles need a heavy blood flow to bring in oxygen and fuel and remove metabolic waste products. Your heart meets this demand by pumping harder and faster.

When you first start exercising, even lightly, there will be a rapid jump in your heart rate. If you continue working at that pace, your heart rate will quickly level off and possibly even drop slightly into what is called steady state. At this point, slight increases in intensity yield slight increases in heart rate in a mostly linear fashion all the way up to maximal effort. Therefore, different percentages of your maximal heart rate will correspond to different percentages of maximal intensity.

How do you determine maximal heart rate? The most accurate way is to have a VO2 max test done in an exercise physiology lab where you run on a treadmill until your heart rate stops increasing. However, that isn't an option for most people so the following equation provides a reasonably good estimate of heart rate max:

HR max = 220 – age in years

For example, if you are 20 years old, your predicted max heart rate would be 200 beats per minute (bpm). Likewise if you are 45, it would be about 175 bpm.

Once you've figured out your max heart rate, then intensities can be quantified as percentages of your max heart rate; the following example is for a 20-year-old:

HR max = 200 bpm

      60% HR max = 120 bpm
      80% HR max = 160 bpm
      90% HR max = 180 bpm

There are three different methods for determining your working heart rate:

1. *Heart rate monitor* – Monitors have a chest strap that you wear under your shirt that detects your pulse and transmits it wirelessly to a watch. Usually it measures and transmits every 10 seconds or so. You just look down at your wrist and there it is.

2. *Heart rate device* – These measurement devices look like a stick with metal handles and a display in the center. You grab the handles, holding the device for 10 to 15 seconds, and it gives you a measurement.

3. *Low-tech counting method* – Find your heart rate using the first and second fingers (the thumb has a pulse of its own and can throw off your count). Press lightly into the wrist until you feel your pulse. Starting at zero, count the number of beats in 15 seconds. You will need a digital watch or clock with a second hand to keep track of the time. Once you have the beats in 15 seconds, multiply that number by 4 to get beats per minute and you're done.

It usually isn't possible to check your pulse during hard exercise. If you are wearing a heart rate monitor, you may be able to glance down occasionally, or if you have a more expensive model, you can set the watch to beep when you go above or below a certain heart rate. If you are using one of the other two methods, you'll have to check it during a rest interval. Start your heart rate check immediately after the work interval because it will drop quickly, especially if you are in good shape. This should give you an idea of how hard you were working during the bout.

Some suggested heart rate target ranges for different intensities of exercise are given below:

- warm-up zone (50–60% HR max)
- low zone (60–80% HR max)
- medium zone (80–90% HR max)
- high zone (90–100% HR max)

Integrating Strength & Conditioning Training

One of the most difficult aspects of strength and conditioning is moving from individual workouts to training programs. How do all of these different types of training methods fit together? When and where should you inject your conditioning workouts, particularly into an ongoing strength training program?

Paired exercises to circuit training progression

The easiest way to start building up your conditioning levels is to reorganize the exercises in your strength program. Nearly all books on lifting stress the importance of resting (sometimes up to 5 minutes) between sets of near-maximal low-rep sets. This leads to a lot of sitting around during heavy lift day. You are likely to get cold and tighten up while sitting around, and the workout will take forever. If you consider rests this long to be necessary, you're most likely lacking in GPP. In other words, you are strong but out of shape.

Rather than spending those rest periods doing nothing, pair your heavy lifts with smaller exercises that won't interfere much with your max performance. Neck work, abdominal and trunk work, and pulling, pressing, or lower-body assistance exercises all work well. For example:

Paired exercises

- bench press – glute ham raise
- incline bench press – calf raise
- overhead press – reverse hypers
- pull-ups – weighted incline sit-ups
- bent over rows – triceps extensions
- high pulls – vertical leg raise
- squats – four-way neck work
- front squats – Russian twist
- deadlifts – internal and external shoulder rotations

The pairs will build conditioning by keeping your heart rate and breathing elevated throughout the workout. You will also get a lot more work done in less time. After a few weeks of training these pairs, increase the conditioning demand by adding in another movement for a three-exercise mini-circuit. It can be another core or assistance exercise or a bodyweight calisthenics drill just to keep your heart rate high. For instance:

Three-exercise mini-circuits

- bench presses – burpees – leg curls
- push presses – bodyweight step-ups – hanging leg raises
- pull-ups – mountain climbers – floor presses
- bent-over rows – jumping jacks – good mornings
- squats – jumping jacks – DB flyes
- deadlifts – in-place high-knee runs – neck bridges

After these mini-circuits, it is a short step to training with full circuits. See the earlier section Circuit Training (page 40) for detailed instructions on setting up circuit workouts. The progression from paired exercises to full circuits is suggested for those athletes who want to ease into circuit training. Starting from scratch with a circuit routine is another option. However, the general fatigue accumulated during such a workout will require a substantially lower training load. If this doesn't bother you, then go for it. If you would prefer to keep your workout poundage up, then use the above progression.

Dedicated conditioning workouts

If you don't want to change your lifting program into a circuit workout or if you want to push your conditioning levels even higher than with circuit work alone, add in separate conditioning workouts to your weekly schedule. The scheduling of your workouts consists of when and how frequently you lift. It is recommended that you keep all strength and conditioning sessions to an hour or less. Otherwise you will not be able to perform at the necessary intensity due to excess fatigue.

When adding conditioning workouts, it is essential to build slowly but consistently in frequency, duration, and intensity. A good guideline is the 2-week rule. This means you increase one of those factors every 2 weeks. Here is a workable conditioning session progression for someone who lifts but does no other conditioning. In this 12-week progression, the duration of the training session refers to the total time of the warm-up and all the training activities.

12-Week Conditioning Workout

Time	Frequency	Duration	Intensity
weeks 1–2	1x per week	25 min.	low to medium
weeks 3–4	2x per week	25 min.	low to medium
weeks 5–6	3x per week	25 min.	low to medium
weeks 7–8	3x per week	25 min.	medium to high
weeks 9–10	3x per week	30 min.	medium to high
weeks 11–12	3x per week	35 min.	medium to high

Delayed Onset Muscle Soreness and Recovery Workouts

One by-product of training that everyone becomes familiar with right away is muscle soreness. During workouts your muscles are damaged. The micro-structural components are stretched and torn, causing an inflammatory response. Like the inflammation from a twisted ankle, this condition leaves your muscles swollen and sore. The phenomenon is called delayed onset muscle soreness (DOMS) because it develops after training and peaks 24 to 48 hours post-exercise. Many people mistakenly attribute this to an accumulation of lactic acid. The lactic acid you build up during a workout can indeed cause a burning pain in your muscles; however, it is quickly buffered and metabolized once you stop.

DOMS is the greatest after a bout of exercise using a new modality or movement or one that emphasizes the eccentric or decelerative component. Thus if you haven't regularly been overhead pressing, training this movement will make you sore even though your previous workouts incorporated other pressing motions. Eccentric work, such as slow negatives, landing from jumps, or running downhill, also tends to cause a great deal of soreness. Take out or minimize the eccentric motion and you also minimize the soreness.

Getting through this soreness is critical if you want to be at your best during the next workout. Although the scientific jury is still out, many top coaches and athletes utilize recovery workouts (or feeder workouts) to help get through soreness more quickly. The premise is that performing low-volume, low-intensity work with the sore muscles in the day or two following the workout can help flush the area with blood. This flushing removes waste products, brings in more nutrients, and helps decrease pain and swelling.

The key to effective recovery work is to keep the intensity and volume low. A couple of low-load, high-rep sets are sufficient. You can incorporate recovery sets into an existing conditioning routine by placing them during rest intervals or at the end of the workout. A dedicated recovery session of 10 to 15 minutes is also a good idea if you have the opportunity. Go through a warm-up, and then mix in some general calisthenics with specific recovery exercises. Finish with static stretching. Here are some examples of effective recovery exercises:

Recovery exercises

- upper body rubber band exercises – presses, pulls, shoulder movements
- MB throws or loading
- pool exercises
- sled dragging
- Indian club swinging
- light KB or DB exercises

Training Journals and Record Keeping

Successful training is the result of a multitude of important factors. The piece that ties them all together, though, is the training journal. A training journal is a workout diary into which each of your workouts is logged. Minimally it contains information about each and every one of your lifting, conditioning, and sports training sessions. The journal can be expanded to include diet, stress levels, supplementation schedules, and other lifestyle factors.

Why is the journal so important?

1. It contains your training plan. If you have not written out some sort of workout program prior to beginning your training, you'll almost certainly spin your wheels and go nowhere. Decide on your training activities for at least the next 12 weeks. Write out the workouts and put them in your journal. Look at the next day's workout in advance so you'll be mentally ready.

2. It contains information about what really happened during the session as opposed to what you had planned. Having a training plan is one thing, but workouts do not always go as planned. What you've written out may be too little, too much, too heavy, or too light. You may miss reps, get sick, have a sprained ankle, or be forced to modify the training on the spot. Having this information will help you tweak your training programs in the future.

3. It lets you know if what you are doing is working. This is potentially the greatest argument for a training journal. Write down all training weights and reps, and the results of any performance testing you do. Compare these numbers to your tests 6 or 12 weeks prior. Did you get stronger or fitter? Where are you compared to 6 months or a year ago? Without writing this information down, you will never remember and will be unable to make such necessary comparisons.

4. It contains information about factors other than your training program that may have influenced your performance. A few late nights and early mornings in a row can really hurt you in the gym. The same is true of work stresses, poor dietary habits, or a cold. If you don't make a note of these circumstances, you might wrongly attribute poor performance to your program rather than to the real cause.

To accomplish the above goals, the training journal should at least have the following information:

- date and time of your workout
- duration of entire workout
- exercises listed in order
- number of sets and repetitions per set
- rest intervals between sets and exercises
- load used on each exercise
- intensity level of the training day
- in general, how you felt before and during the workout

Additional information that will help diagnose any sudden increases or decreases in performance may be added:

- amount and quality of sleep the previous night
- any injuries, aches, or pains you had coming into the workout
- last thing you had to eat before the workout and when you had it
- any stimulants (caffeine or ephedra) you had in your system
- unusual circumstances, such as a fight with your spouse, bad day at work, or drinking binge the night before

It is useful to include dietary information both for the acute effect eating patterns might have on performance (such as low or high blood sugar) and for the longer-term goal of gaining muscle or reducing body fat. Useful dietary information includes:

- time of meal or snack
- portion size of each food
- calorie/fat/protein information, if known

The supplement industry is a booming business, and chances are that if you don't currently take some sort of supplement, you will experiment at some point. People have mixed feelings about nutritional supplementation, and I don't intend to argue for or against it in this book. However, if you decide to use one or more supplements, it would be helpful to know if they actually worked for you or not. Why spend your money and get no benefit? You would also want to know if they were hindering your performance. By making notes of what you are taking, when you take it, and in what dose, you are in a position to evaluate a supplement's value. If the supplement is supposed to boost your strength, did your numbers go up? If it is supposed to increase endurance, were you able to run longer, harder, or farther? Although this method is not scientific in the strictest sense, it is the best objective method available for you to decide what works. When adding nutritional supplements, be sure to add them one at a time. If you start taking 12 different pills and powders at once, there is no way to tell which work and which do not.

Aside from workout information, your journal is a place you can write down your short- and long-term training goals. Goal-setting is an important part of any conditioning program. Read back over these goals regularly to cement them into your mind. Always keep your eye on the prize. Include motivational quotes that you read or hear. Sometimes repeating a short, inspiring quote as a sort of mantra is all you need to get you through a seemingly impossible workout. Finally, cut out pictures of your heroes and paste them in the journal. When you see these athletes in the midst of competition or training, you'll know that they had to sweat and bleed just like you to get where they are.

Overtraining

Overtraining is what happens when you do too much training and/or have too little recovery. This can be summarized by the General Adaptation Syndrome (GAS) of physiologist Hans Selye. GAS has three stages:

1. *Alarm* – This is the stage in which the body is presented with stress. It responds in an attempt to maintain homeostasis.
2. *Resistance* – In this stage, the body makes adjustments to a repeated stress so that it is better able to adapt during the alarm stage.
3. *Exhaustion* – Chronic stress overcomes the body's ability to deal with it and it breaks down, resulting in injury or illness.

Selye originally proposed this model as a method of describing the immune function, but it can be applied to any stress. Thus, the development of antibodies to viral infection and increased heart-pumping capacity due to conditioning operate on the same principle. The key to proper training and recovery lies in balancing the stress you place on your body and the recovery time allowed for it to develop resistance. Exhaustion is synonymous with overtraining. Overtraining is defined as a syndrome or a collection of clustered symptoms. Taken alone, none of these symptoms is enough to diagnose a state of overtraining. However, if several are present at the same time, it may be necessary to adjust your training schedule:

Symptoms of overtraining

- Elevated heart rate in the morning – to use this measure, you need a baseline morning pulse rate
- Excessive or persistent soreness – again, this must be over and above what you would expect from hard training
- Physical burnout – a constant feeling of tiredness and lethargy
- Mental burnout – a big drop in your motivation to train
- Drop in performance – a sudden decrease in your ability to perform to your normal capacity during training or competition
- Insomnia – inability to sleep
- Mood swings – depression, irritability, or nervousness
- Illness – getting a cold or virus or getting one of them more frequently due to depressed immune function
- Headaches – tension headaches or migraines
- Excessive thirst or hunger – eating more than normal or a seeming inability to get full
- Loss of appetite – lack of hunger throughout the day even though you haven't eaten much
- Overuse injury – shin splints, tendonitis, or bursitis could mean too much repetitive stress on one area

Many of these symptoms could be indicative of serious illness and not just overtraining. Before you make any modifications to your training program, see a doctor to make sure that you are otherwise healthy. If nothing else is wrong and you have a few of these symptoms, it is likely that you are overtrained. Dealing with overtraining can be difficult. Stopping exercise entirely until you bounce back is simply not an option for hardcore trainees or competitive athletes.

Here is one reasonable plan for getting yourself back on track:

1. Take 2 to 3 days off completely from training. Go for walks and stretch but do not do anything too physically demanding.

2. Build back up to your pre-overtraining level over the course of 3 to 4 weeks. Drop the intensity, frequency, and duration back down. Make sure your workouts, especially for the first week, leave you feeling hardly worked out. Consider this to be maintenance training while your body recovers.

3. Cut out as much non-workout related stress as possible for this month. Be sure to eat properly and get a lot of sleep.

Now that you're back to where you were, the next step is to analyze why you ended up overtrained and how to avoid it in the future. Typically overtraining occurs after a dramatic increase in training volume or during periods of stress. When family, work, or school puts additional stress on you, lighten up a bit on your workouts to compensate.

Sport-specific Conditioning Programs

What if you aren't just training for all-around fitness, but trying to get in the best shape to play your sport(s) of choice? How do you go about designing an effective training program? The first step is to conduct what is known as a needs analysis, in which you look at the typical intensity, duration, and type of activity the sport involves. The needs analysis will give you insight into what energy systems and muscle groups you should emphasize in your training program.

Needs Analysis

1. What is the length of a game or match?

2. How is the game or match divided? Is it one continuous bout of moderate-intensity work, as in a 10K run, or is it broken up into a series of high-intensity bouts with rest periods between? Is it a short, maximal effort sprint?

3. Will there be a single match or will you have several matches in a tournament? How long do you have between them to recover?

4. What is the dominant mode of exercise in your sport? Is it running, swimming, grappling with an opponent, or something else? Are there multiple modes?

5. Which muscle groups are most used during your sport? Is it primarily a pushing, pulling, or lower-body activity?

Let's take boxing, for example, to see step by step how to perform a needs analysis. First, boxing fights vary in length depending on whether the athlete is collegiate, amateur, or pro. Most commonly they are 3 minutes long and separated by a 1-minute rest period. The boxer must be able to keep a near maximal pace for as many 3-minute rounds as are required in a fight in case it goes the distance. If you watch a boxing match closely, the action is broken. A fighter will move and dance around, looking for an opening in his opponent's defense, and then come in with one or more combos. After the flurry, the boxers will separate or clinch, allowing some rest. The work done in boxing is very specific to the sport. You must incorporate punching, blocking, defensive moves, and footwork into your conditioning workouts. The arms, shoulders, core, and lower legs should receive the greatest emphasis due to their importance in the sport.

Sample Needs Analysis: Boxing

Duration	5 x 3 min. (60 sec. rest)
Intensity	short 5–30 sec. high-intensity bouts with low/moderate intensity work in between
Mode/muscles	boxing specific skills, arm, shoulder, core, and leg endurance

After you have done the needs analysis, you can begin to select appropriate conditioning activities for the boxer and to prioritize them. Based on the analysis, the amount of training time could be split up as follows:

75% high intensity
- short maximal intervals (20 to 60 seconds) with brief rests
- boxing drills, jump rope, sprints, calisthenics, DB/KB exercises, sandbags, etc.

15% moderate intensity
- longer, continuous intensity rounds (90 seconds to 5 minutes) with rests between
- boxing drills, jump rope, runs, MB circuits, BB/DB complexes, etc.

10% low intensity
- longer duration (15 to 20 minutes) continuous work for aerobic base
- running, swimming, rowing, jumping rope, etc.

After you have decided on a percentage breakdown for your sport, divide the total weekly training time up into different intensity zones. You can split them up over the course of the week or use all three zones in a single session. Fatigue will affect higher-intensity work to a greater degree than lower-intensity work. It is therefore advisable to perform a session's activities in order of descending intensity.

Sport-Specific Conditioning Needs Analysis

Adapted from Fox and Matthews' *Interval Training* (1974)

Sport	% emphasis on energy system training		
	Phosphagen	Glycolytic	Oxidative
Baseball	80	20	-
Basketball	85	15	-
Fencing	90	10	-
Field hockey	60	20	20
Football	90	10	-
Golf	95	5	-
Gymnastics	90	10	-
Ice hockey			
forwards, defense	80	20	-
goalie	95	5	-
Lacrosse			
goalie, defense, attack men	80	20	-
midfielders, man-down	60	20	20
Rowing	20	30	50
Skiing			
slalom, jumping, downhill	80	20	-
cross country	-	5	95
pleasure skiing	34	33	33
Soccer			
goalie, wings, strikers	80	20	-
halfbacks, link men	60	20	20
Swimming and diving			
50 yd., diving	98	2	-
100 yd.	80	15	5
200 yd.	30	65	5
400, 500 yd.	20	40	40
1500, 1650 yd.	10	20	70
Tennis	70	20	10
Track and field			
100, 220 yd.	98	2	-
field events	90	10	-
440 yd.	80	15	5
880 yd.	30	65	5
1 mi.	20	55	25
2 mi.	20	40	40
3 mi.	10	20	70
6 mi. (cross-country)	5	15	80
marathon	-	5	95
Volleyball	90	10	-
Wrestling	90	10	-

Mouthpieces and conditioning work

If you wear a mouthpiece during your event (the case in most contact sports), then you should wear it any time you lift or do conditioning work. Any type of mouthpiece will restrict your breathing to some degree. The time to get used to the effect it will have on your conditioning is during training, not competition. A good idea is to wear a double (upper and lower) mouthpiece during your workouts, even if you compete in a single. This will make it feel even easier to get air during your competitions.

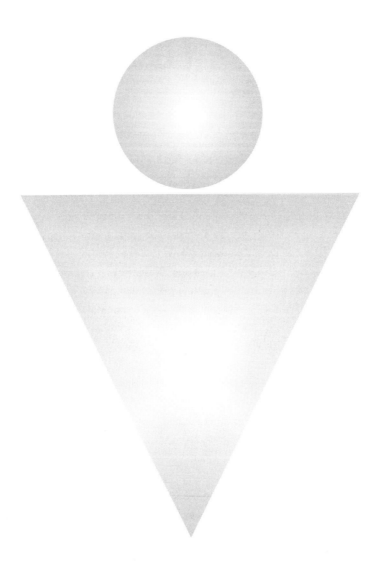

Chapter 3

Training Modalities

$\mathbf{T}$his chapter gives a very broad overview of various training modalities that work well for conditioning. It's likely that many of these will be familiar to you; however, just as many will probably be new. Often, when presented with a new type of training, a coach or athlete will fixate upon it at the expense of everything else. Avoid succumbing to such narrow-minded faddishness. There are no secret weapons in strength and conditioning except determination and hard work. My suggestion is to try everything. Ignore the marketing hype and give any new training programs or workouts a fair but thorough evaluation. If you are a coach, make sure you try them out yourself before you teach or make your athletes do them. If you can't learn the proper technique in a single session, don't expect your athletes to do so as well.

Some important questions to ask about any new modality are:

1. Does this modality do what it says it will do? Does the rationale make logical sense based on your training experience?
2. Is there any research to support it or other methods like it?
3. Have any top coaches or athletes (other than those paid to endorse it) used this modality successfully?
4. Does it appear safe?
5. Is it appropriate for you or your athletes or is it better suited to those more or less trained?
6. How difficult to teach or learn are the techniques involved?
7. Do you have the equipment and facilities necessary to implement the modality? If not, do the benefits it will provide appear to be worth the cost?

Think of each method as a tool in your toolbox. All are appropriate in certain circumstances. Some tools you will use regularly and some only occasionally. A wide variety of training methods will keep you or your athletes excited about training and mentally involved. It is very easy to slip into a rut and simply go through the motions—sometimes all that is needed to break through training plateaus is to mix things up a bit.

Medicine Balls

The medicine ball has been a staple of athletic training for years. Almost every older gym has a few battered leather balls stashed away in a corner. In recent years there has been a revived interest in medicine ball training and a multitude of new designs have hit the market. You can now find ones intended to bounce or not bounce, to roll or not roll. Some are small enough to simulate a baseball while others are large enough to mimic the stones lifted in strongman competitions. My advice is to pick up two or three general-purpose balls designed to absorb a lot of dropping and throwing abuse. Later, if you want to experiment with some more specialized applications, invest in the other designs.

Many of the exercises performed with the medicine ball could theoretically be done with weights or dumbbells. The advantage of the balls is that 1) they allow you to do throws and drops in an indoor setting, and 2) they are more forgiving if you hit yourself or your workout partner. The exercises in the following section work extremely well in circuits. Because medicine ball training means working with a low load and without an eccentric component in many of the throwing exercises, they make a great off-day training modality.

Loading basic exercises

When you need a lighter portable load for basic upper- and lower-body exercises, medicine balls are ideal. Hold the medicine ball in various positions for squats, lunges, step-ups, running, or abdominal work. Presses and rows can also be done at various angles in a supine, seated, or standing position. Medicine balls have traditionally been used to add weight to abdominal and other core movements and work very well for that purpose.

Partner and rebounder passes

Medicine ball passes can be done either with a training partner or with a medicine ball rebounder, a sort of mini-trampoline. Passes work the entire upper body, particularly the shoulder girdle and trunk. In addition, high repetitions of even a light weight will tax your cardiovascular system. When doing any of the following throws, you can either do most of the work with your arms, or keep your arms almost straight and throw more from the trunk. Vary the way you throw the ball from rep to rep or set to set. When catching the ball, allow your shoulders and core to give a bit to help decelerate the load and protect your joints.

Here are some of the many variations of the medicine ball pass:

- overhead pass – straight overhead or at 45-degree angles
- push or chest pass – straight from the chest, straight out to the side, or angled up or down
- scoop pass – between or beside the legs; or throw straight ahead, straight up, or over the back

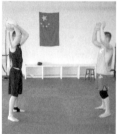 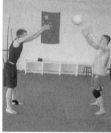 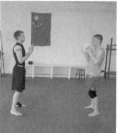 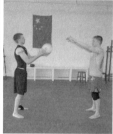

Medicine ball overhead pass.　　　　Medicine ball chest pass.

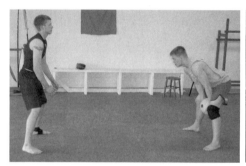 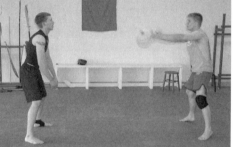

Medicine ball scoop pass.

After you've practiced the basic passes above, you can mix up your routine by using some of the following variations:

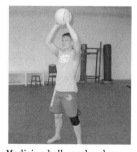

- stance variations – use a wide, narrow, single-leg, or low-lunge position
- moving throws – rather than standing in place, walk or jog with your partner while passing the ball back and forth
- squats or lunges – incorporate a squat or lunge as you throw or catch the ball

Medicine ball overhead press.

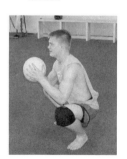 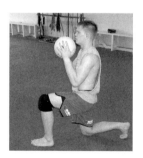

Medicine ball squat.　　　Medicine ball lunge.

Slams and distance throws

If you have a sturdy medicine ball that will not roll or bounce excessively after impact, you can do some different types of throwing. Slams are throws done for maximum power at a close target. Lifting the ball up overhead and throwing it to the ground as hard as possible is an example. These are well-suited for athletes who have limited space or who want to do more consecutive reps without having to chase the ball.

Distance throws require a larger area and you propel the medicine ball for maximum distance and/or height. As with partner and rebounder throws, you can vary the muscular emphasis by throwing more with the arms or trunk, or by changing the amount of leg movement. Many variations of these types of exercises are possible:

* throw from overhead to the ground
* push throw at a wall or for distance
* rotational throw at a wall or for distance
* overhead back throw at a wall or for distance
* diagonal overhead back throw at a wall or for distance

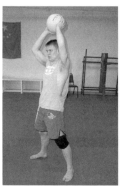 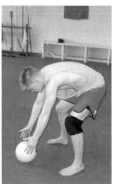 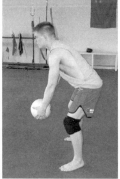 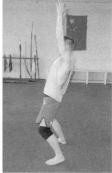

Medicine ball floor slam.   Medicine ball overhead back throw for distance.

Sandbags and Heavybags

Heavy sandbags are a very low-tech way to make some substantial gains in strength and endurance. Unlike barbells and dumbbells, the weight inside the bag shifts, making it much more difficult to lift. With no ready handles, you just hug a sandbag or grab a handful of the material, which provides an excellent grip workout. Sandbags are particularly effective for football and rugby players, judoka, wrestlers, and fighters who must control a resisting opponent. Heavybags detached from their hanging chains can be used as makeshift bags and are more durable for throwing exercises.

Carries and drags

Carrying a sandbag using a variety of holding positions is an excellent way to improve endurance while working the upper body and core isometrically. You can hold the bag on one or two shoulders, like a suitcase, in a Zercher squat position, or in many other ways. Each position provides a unique challenge. During the carry, maintain the same grip the entire time or rotate positions as upper-body fatigue sets in. Drags can be performed by gripping the bag or attaching it to a rope, cable, or chain and moving forward, sideways, or backward. Carry or drag the bag for a specified distance or time interval. The heavier the bag is, the shorter the distance or interval. Distances as short as 20 feet and as long as one-half mile or so can be used, depending on your goals. For more information about sandbag training, see my book *The Complete Sandbag Training Course*.

Pressing

All barbell pressing motions can be mimicked with a sandbag. The instability provides an added challenge, as the bag will tend to sag in the middle as it is pressed. The drooping bag forces you to squeeze it together as you press, increasing the demands on the pectorals and shoulder stabilizer muscles. Some common exercises include bench presses, incline presses, floor presses, and overhead presses.

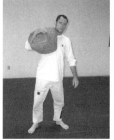

Sandbag one-shoulder hold.

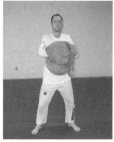

Bear hug hold with sandbag.

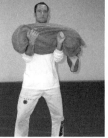

Sandbag Zercher hold.

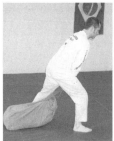

Forward drag with sandbag.

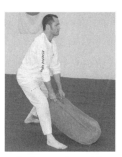

Backward drag with sandbag.

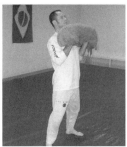
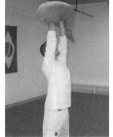

Overhead press.

Pulling

Barbell pulling motions also work well with sandbags. The difference is in the intense work your hands and forearms will get from gripping the bag material, which requires a reduced load relative to your normal barbell workouts. Excellent options for pulling work include bent-over rows, upright rows, shrugs, and curls.

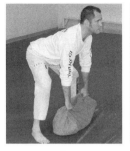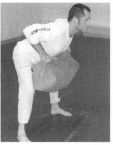

Bent-over rows with sandbag.

Lower-body exercises

With sandbags, squats are still the king of exercises. You can hold the bag any number of ways, such as on one shoulder or two shoulders, overhead,

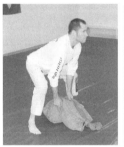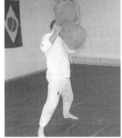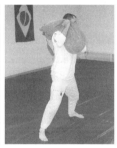

Shouldering a sandbag.

or in a bear hug. In addition to squats, lunges, step-ups, and deadlifts are all excellent conditioning movements. The instability of the bag will provide extra core work as you rev up your heart rate and train your anaerobic endurance.

Olympic-style and power movements

Many Olympic lifting exercises can be performed using the bag. Cleans, push presses, push jerks, and shouldering the bag in one motion from the floor all build power and explosiveness in addition to endurance. The form on these lifts is a bit freer than with a barbell or dumbbells because the bag will shift in the air and during the catch. Start with a lighter bag and practice the form before using heavier loads. Sandbag snatches could injure the shoulder and are not recommended.

Throwing the bag is truly a full-body workout. However, throws can damage your sandbag and cause it to rupture. When throwing, it is best to use a heavy bag with the chains removed. Throw the bag forward with a push, backward over your head, sideways with a twisting motion, or any other way you can manage. These exercises can be done for distance, reps, or time. For distance work, throw the bag as far as possible, run to it, and repeat for the specified distance. To progress, try to cover the same distance with fewer and fewer throws.

Turkish get-ups

The Turkish get-up is one of the best all-around strength and conditioning exercises there is. It is especially useful for combat athletes because it mimics moving around an

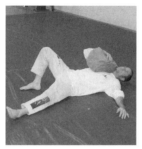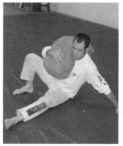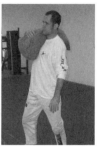

Turkish get-up with sandbag, floor to standing.

opponent. There are two different versions. For the first, start in a standing position, with the bag draped over one shoulder. Go down on one knee and then lie back until you are completely supine. Keeping the bag securely on your shoulder, come back to a full standing position by reversing the movement: sit up, post your free hand on the ground, and then bring your feet underneath you. Do an equal number of reps with the bag on the left and right shoulders. To perform the second version, start by holding the bag in the Zercher position in front of your body. Squat down and lie all the way down. Come all the way back to standing without letting the bag touch the ground.

Agility Work

Agility work is common in sports training; however, anyone can benefit from basic agility drills. They are an essential part of GPP work and are a recommended method of conditioning when performed in extended sets. It is best to perform tumbling or jumping exercises on a mat or a relatively soft surface to avoid injury. Be sure to practice and become proficient in the technique of each drill before performing it to the point of fatigue.

Tumbling

Tumbling refers to basic floor gymnastics and falling. I'm not talking about the high skill movements that gymnasts do in competitive routines but fundamental falls, rolls, cartwheels, and roundoffs. These skills teach body control, balance, and kinesthetic awareness, and those who cannot currently perform them will improve their athleticism tremendously by learning how. The falling techniques are taken from judo training where they are called *ukemi waza*. Judo training involves a lot of throwing, and proper landing is essential for safety as well as for being a good training partner.

To learn the falling and rolling techniques, start by practicing them in a seated position. As your skill improves, begin from a low squatting position and eventually from a standing start.

It is helpful to have a spotter assist you if you have never done cartwheels or roundoffs before. Some of the rolling techniques can make you dizzy, particularly at first. If you incorporate these exercises into a mixed modal circuit or workout, be sure to give your head time to stop spinning before attempting any high-skill exercise such as cleans or snatches.

- **Back fall**

  Begin the back fall by crossing your arms on your chest and tucking your chin. Squat down and fall on your back, allowing your legs to come up and back. Slap the mat with both hands, palms down, and exhale when you hit. If your chin is not tucked, your head may hit the mat and give you a concussion. Reaching for the ground rather than smacking the mat as your back hits can result in a damaged shoulder, wrist, or elbow. Holding your breath on impact can knock the wind out of you.

- **Side fall**

  The starting position for the side fall is standing with one foot forward. Swing your back leg across your body, squat down, and fall onto your side. Slap the mat with one hand and keep the other on your chest. As in the back fall, it is important to tuck your chin and exhale as you land.

- **Front fall**

  For the front fall, squat down, kick your feet out behind you, and fall forward, landing on your palms, forearms, and balls of your feet; your head, chest, and legs should remain off the mat. Your feet should be wider than shoulder-width apart. A variation of this fall can be done without supporting the body on the toes. Allow your whole body to hit at the same time so that you distribute the force over as large an area as possible. Keep your elbows tucked under you so that you can use your palms and forearms to prevent your head from hitting the mat.

- **Forward somersault roll**

  Tuck your chin, squat down, put your hands on the floor, and roll straight over. Keep your body tucked throughout the roll. Return to a standing position and repeat. Keep your chin tucked as tightly as possible to prevent neck injury. Once this basic position is mastered, the roll can be combined with a vertical jump to increase the endurance demands and build explosiveness.

- **Forward shoulder roll**

  In the forward shoulder roll, you go over one shoulder rather than both as in the somersault roll. Start in a staggered stance, with one foot leading. As you go forward, tuck your chin and initiate floor contact with the blade of your hand (outside of your pinky finger). Continue rolling over, landing on your side in a side-fall position. Alternatively, you could continue the roll and come to a standing position.

- **Backward somersault roll**

  The body position for the back somersault roll is the same as for the front roll, but it is typically a bit more difficult to master the backward motion. Keep your chin and body tightly tucked during the roll. If your knees come away from your chest mid-roll, you'll have difficulty finishing it. After you have mastered the basic roll, you can add an extension at the end: just as you are completing the roll, kick your feet straight, press off with your arms, and end standing up.

- **Backward shoulder roll**

  Squat down, stretch your arms out straight, and roll back over one shoulder. You must move your head away from the shoulder you roll over to open up the proper space. Be careful not to roll straight over your neck. Come up to a squatting or standing position and repeat.

- **Diving forward rolls**

  After you have mastered forward rolling, you can increase the difficulty and conditioning effect by diving forward into the roll. Start conservatively, gradually increasing the height or distance of the jump. Hurdles, boxes, or kneeling training partners can be used to set the distance or height.

- **Cartwheels and roundoffs**

  Cartwheels and roundoffs are both basic gymnastics skills that can typically be learned with a few weeks of consistent practice. Start with the cartwheel. The idea is to make a complete sideways rotation with your body, starting on your hands, keeping the legs straight up in the air, and landing back on your feet; your chest is vertical during the movement. Common problems are bending at the waist and allowing the legs to cross over one another upon landing. The key is to get full handstand extension, tighten the core, and push off with the arms as you finish.

  It is a short step to the roundoff once you've learned the cartwheel. In mid-cartwheel, use your abdominals to twist your body around and land facing opposite from the way that you started. Both of these exercises take some practice and can be learned more easily with the help of a spotter to guide you through the movements until you get a feel for them.

- **Tumbling combos**

  After you've become proficient at the basic tumbling exercises, you can begin to string them together to increase the cardiovascular demands. Here are some example combinations that flow well:

  - left forward shoulder roll – right forward shoulder roll to standing – back fall
  - forward somersault roll with jump – back somersault roll with extension
  - right roundoff into right backward shoulder roll – left roundoff into left backward shoulder roll
  - backward somersault roll with extension – front fall

Jumping

Jumps are fundamental movement skills that build strength, power, and endurance throughout the lower body. Jumping drills can be classified into either quick or power types. Quick jumps are rapid and repetitive and involve mostly the muscles of the foot and lower leg. The emphasis is on minimizing ground contact time. In power jumping, the goal is to achieve maximal height or distance on each rep. To boost the intensity of moving jump drills, perform them on an incline or up stairs.

Quick jumps

Quick jumps are performed similar to jumping rope. The idea is to come off the ground as quickly as possible but just high enough to leave the ground. Speed is the key. When quick jumps are performed with forward, backward, or lateral movement, the distance covered on each jump is short. It is useful, although not necessary, to mark the landing spots on the floor using tape. These marks will give you a target and keep your jumping distances even. Low obstacles such as sticks, short hurdles, or cones may also be used to ensure a minimum jump height.

The following jumps can be performed double-footed or single-footed, or with an alternating foot pattern:

Stationary jumps

- front to back – hop about 12 inches forward, then back to the original position
- side to side – hop about 12 inches to the left and then back to the right
- diagonal – hop toward your right front corner, and then back to the start; complete all the reps, then repeat on the other side
- four corners – hop on the corners of a marked (or imaginary) square; for even development, do an equal number of reps starting left and right
- shuffle splits – start in a front lunge position. Jump into the air and switch legs to land in a lunge position on the other side. You can use shallow lunges and go faster, or deeper lunges and go slower

Moving jumps

- linear jumps – hop in a straight line forward or backward
- lateral jumps – hop to the left or right
- zigzag jumps – hop diagonally to the left, then to the right, going forward or backward
- pattern jumps – follow a specified pattern of dots or lines on the floor; these can incorporate many variations and direction changes

Power jumps

Power jumps require maximal effort on each rep. Your goal is to cover as much distance as possible (horizontally or laterally) with each jump. Due to this increased intensity, power jumping volume must be much lower than quick jumps. It is also very important to warm up thoroughly before performing these exercises. Several short series of quick jumps make great warm-ups for power jumps. When landing from a high or long jump, be sure to decelerate properly by bending your knees so that the shock will not harm your joints. All of these exercises can be performed either single- or double-footed.

- vertical jump – squat down, stop and pause for 2 seconds, then jump has high as possible, reaching upward with your arms
- countermovement* vertical jump – dip down into a squatting position, allowing your arms to swing backward, then immediately burst up into a vertical jump
- broad jump – squat down, stop and pause for 2 seconds, then jump as far forward as possible
- countermovement* broad jump – dip down into a squatting position, allowing your arms to swing backward, then immediately jump as far forward as possible
- lateral broad jump – squat down, stop and pause for 2 seconds, then jump as far to the left or right as possible
- countermovement* lateral broad jump – squat down and immediately spring up, jumping as far to the left or right as possible
- obstacle jumps – do any of the above over obstacles or using areas marked on the floor or wall to ensure a minimum distance or height

*In a countermovement jump, you dip down and spring up quickly out of a partial squatting position. In the broad jump, you do this to cover horizontal distance, instead of jumping straight up.

- box jumps – perform a vertical jump onto a box or other stable surface
- frog jumps – squat down on your toes and jump forward, landing in the same position
- tuck jumps – jump as high as possible and pull your knees to your chest when you are in the air
- star jumps – jump as high as possible and extend both arms and legs out as far as you can
- depth jumps – step off a box onto both feet, then immediately jump for maximal height or distance. Depth jumps are plyometric exercises and can be very stressful to the joints if you are not prepared. It is essential to have a base level of lower-body strength (squat 1RM of at least your bodyweight) before adding these to your workout. Depth jumps are maximal attempts, so the sets and repetitions must be kept low: 4 or 5 sets of 5 or fewer reps are plenty in one workout. Rest your legs for a minute or so between sets and never perform depth jumps to failure

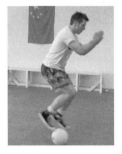 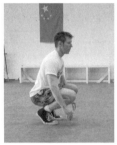 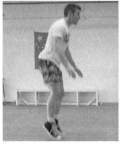 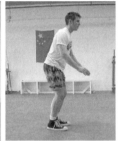

Obstacle jump.   Frog jump.

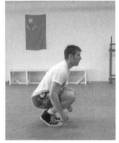 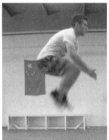 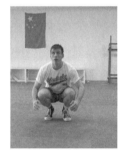 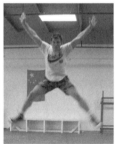

Tuck jump.   Star jump.

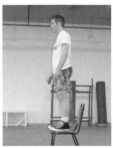 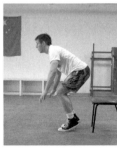 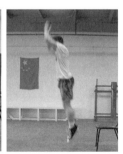

Depth jump.

Agility Ladders, Runs, and Drills

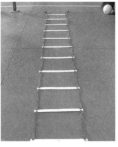

Agility ladders

Agility ladders are standard training tools for field and court sports and are readily available from athletic supply companies that cater to those athletes. It is also easy to make one yourself, using rope and short pieces of thin PVC pipe as the rungs. Typically ladders come in 15- to 20-foot lengths and can be laid next to one another for longer drills or placed in different patterns, such as squares or diamonds.

Agility ladder.

The following are some of the more common patterns with agility ladders:

- high-knee single hit – bring your knees up high on each step and stay on your toes. Step only once inside each rung. Run forward, backward, or sideways
- high-knee double hit – bring your knees up high on each step and stay on your toes. Step twice (once with each foot) inside each rung. Run forward, backward, or sideways
- in and out – facing the side of the agility ladder, move one foot into a rung then out, then move the other foot in and out, move on to the next rung and continue; run left or right
- jumping – most of the moving quick jump exercises covered in the jumping section may be done with an agility ladder
- two in and two out – run forward, hitting once with each foot inside the rung then once with each foot outside the ladder. You can also do this backward
- 90-degree hop – start facing forward with one foot in and one out of the first rung. Jump and turn 90 degrees so that one foot is in the first rung and one in the second and you are facing to the side. Jump and turn 90 degrees so that you are facing forward with one foot in and one out of the second rung

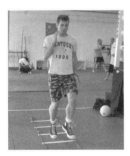
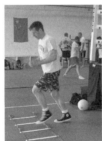
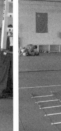
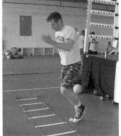
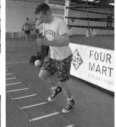

High-knee single
hit pattern.

In and out pattern.

Agility ladder workouts are typically designed so that you do a specific number of runs down the ladder as a set. Ladder runs fit well into circuits as a form of active rest between upper-body exercises. Another possibility is to set a time to perform rounds of ladder runs. Set up a sequence of running patterns and repeat them with minimal rest until the round is up.

Agility runs

Agility running uses something other than standard running form to work agility or specific muscle groups. Work at a moderate pace on these until you get the movement down and then speed up:

- backward runs – jog with normal technique but move backward
- high-knee – bring your knees up as high as possible on each step; run forward, backward, or sideways
- glute kicks – bring your feet up as high as you can behind you and kick yourself in the rear on each step; move forward, backward, or sideways
- Carioca step – move to the left, stepping in front of your left foot with your right, then behind your left foot with your right; do this left and right

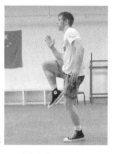 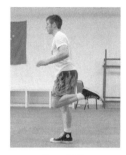

High-knee run.   Glute kick.

- slide shuffle – slide your trailing foot up to your lead foot, then slide your lead foot ahead. Move sideways using this motion and keep your stance low

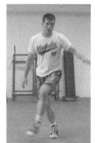 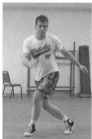 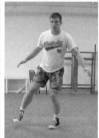 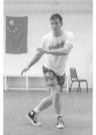 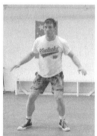

Carioca step.

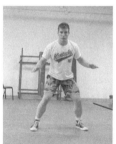 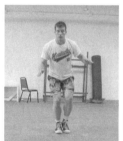 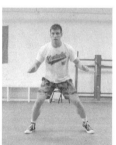

Slide shuffle.

Do agility runs on a track or around your training room. Mix up the foot patterns as you work all areas of your lower body. Use these exercises in addition to runs when between exercise stations in circuits or obstacle courses.

Hurdles

Hurdles are an excellent way to condition the lower body and build dynamic flexibility in the hips, an essential attribute for almost all sports. Hurdles come in two basic types, mini hurdles and high hurdles. Mini hurdles can be used as obstacles for low-amplitude jumps or for running patterns in much the same way as an agility ladder. For this reason, we will limit our discussion to the unique drills that can be performed using high hurdles. High hurdles can be purchased from an athletic supply company or constructed using lengths of PVC pipe. Although many drills can be done using only one or two hurdles, it is ideal to have at least four hurdles so that several repetitions can be performed in a single linear set:

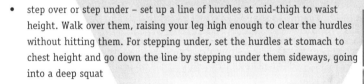

- stiff-leg over – facing the end of the hurdle, swing one leg up and over with minimal knee bend. As the up leg completes its movement, you bounce or skip sideways slightly to the next hurdle, and repeat. Perform these along a series of hurdles and do an equal number of reps swinging your leg from the outside in and the inside out. The height of the hurdle will depend on your flexibility, but waist height is a good guideline

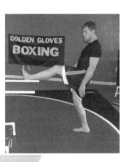

Stiff-leg over.

- fire hydrant walk – start with the hurdles to your right side. Step forward with your left leg, and then bring your right leg up and over the hurdle in a semi-circular motion. Set the hurdles at a manageable height based on your flexibility

- step over or step under – set up a line of hurdles at mid-thigh to waist height. Walk over them, raising your leg high enough to clear the hurdles without hitting them. For stepping under, set the hurdles at stomach to chest height and go down the line by stepping under them sideways, going into a deep squat

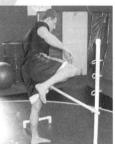

Fire hydrant.

- step over and under – set up the hurdles in a line, alternating a lower hurdle (mid-thigh to waist height) with a higher hurdle (stomach to chest height). Step over the low hurdles and step under the high ones. To step under, face sideways and go into a deep squat. Try not to hit any of the hurdles

- jump over and step under – this is an advanced exercise that is extremely fatiguing. Jump over a waist-high hurdle, land, turn, and immediately step under it. Move as fast as possible without knocking over the hurdle

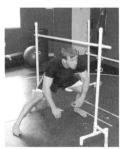

Step under.

Cone drills

Cone drills are commonly used to teach running and cutting patterns in court and field sports, but they also make interesting and demanding conditioning activities for any athlete. Use high-visibility cones that collapse when stepped on to ensure safety. Some different ways that cones can be used include:

- linear sprinting drills – set up the cones at specified distances from one another. The distance between the cones is used to quantify work and rest intervals or to tell you when to switch exercises. For instance, you could sprint from cone 1 to cone 2, jog from cone 2 to cone 3, and then sprint from cone 3 to cone 4.

  Alternatively you could sprint from cone 1 to cone 2, high-knee sprint from cone 2 to cone 3, and then lunge walk from cone 3 to cone 4. All types of moving exercises, including hopping, bear crawls, and tumbling, may be used

- directional change drills – set up the cones in specified patterns to practice quick changes of direction. A square pattern might require a sprint up one side, a quick slide shuffle across the top, a backpedal down the opposite side, and then a slide shuffle back to the start.

- obstacles – set up the cones to be jumped over or run around when doing, for example, in-place hops; multiple cones may be set up in series to make the course more challenging

When using agility exercises for conditioning, you can apply a sets and reps format, adding either sets or reps over the course of several workouts as a method of progression. You might also use a given distance rather than a specific number of reps. As your conditioning improves, gradually increase the distance to be covered. Cones make great station markers for circuits and obstacle course workouts.

Dot drills

Dot drills are another standard agility exercise that can really give your lower body a work-out. The concept is very simple. First, paint, draw, or mark out with tape a grid or other pattern of circles on the floor. The training area will look much like a game of Twister. Dot drill mats are also available for purchase if you don't want to make your own. Next, decide on a repetitive stepping pattern, using the dots as guides. The effect is similar to the agility ladder except that you don't actually move down the floor, which makes dot drills great for those with little training space. Perform the stepping patterns for reps or continuously for timed intervals.

When designing the stepping patterns consider the following options:

- single- and double-footed steps
- forward, backward, and diagonal steps
- single- and double-footed jumps
- jumps with a 90- or 180-degree turn

Bodyweight Exercises

Learning to control your own bodyweight is a prerequisite for athletic success. Bodyweight and partner exercises require almost no equipment and very little space, making them ideal for conditioning circuits, home workouts, or workouts while traveling. Most of these exercises can be adjusted to make them more or less difficult; however, if you are a relatively new trainee or have a high bodyweight, it may be impossible for you to complete more than a few reps of some movements. It is recommended that you reserve these for your heavier lifting days so that they don't interfere with your recovery.

Weight vests are a great way to increase the difficulty of bodyweight exercises. Vests typically come in 20- or 40-lb. adjustable varieties. When adding a weight vest, never start with the maximum weight your vest will accommodate, particularly when performing jumps. Add 5 lb. or so, moving up gradually over a period of weeks. Even with a slight increase in weight, you'll feel a difference in your heart rate and respiration.

Full-body Exercises

Jumping jacks – these can be done in the standard manner or by using one of these variations:

- seal jump – bring your arms across the front of your body and touch your palms on each rep
- Highlander – cross your arms in front of your body and your feet over one another on each rep
- shuffle split – bring one foot forward into a staggered stance on each rep, alternating feet

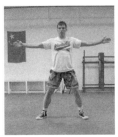 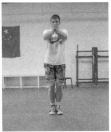 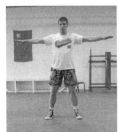 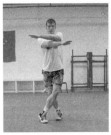

Seal jump.   Highlander jump.

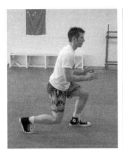 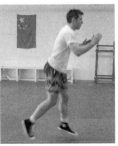 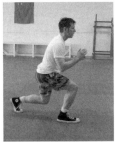

Shuffle split jump.

Mountain climber – get into push-up position, with one leg extended and the other pulled in toward your chest. In one motion bring your extended leg in to your chest and extend your tucked leg so that you are in the same position on the opposite side. Repeat for the specified number of reps.

- double-footed – instead of the alternating leg running motion, jump both feet up to your chest at the same time and then back

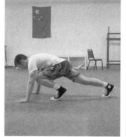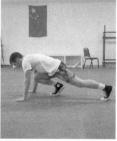

Mountain climber.

Squat thrust – start in a standing position. Squat down, put both hands on the floor, and jump your feet out into push up position. Jump your feet back in and stand up.

- bodybuilder – an extended version of the squat thrust, it is done on an 8-count:
  1) squat down, 2) jump your feet into push-up position, 3) jump your legs wide apart, 4) jump them back together, 5) descend into a push-up, 6) return to push-up position, 7) jump your feet back in, and 8) stand up
- burpee – this is a squat thrust with a jump as you stand up. You can do it in place with a vertical jump or moving by using a forward, sideways, or backward broad jump
- dumbbell – any of these squat thrust variations can be done while holding a pair of dumbbells to increase the resistance

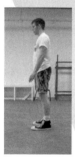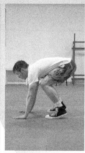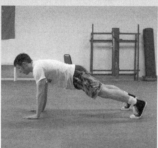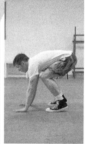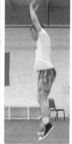

Burpee.

Squats – these can be done in traditional flat-footed style or using one of many possible variations:

- stance – move the stress to different muscle groups by using narrow, medium, or wide stances
- Hindu squat – this popular version begins with descending into a squat with your arms at your sides. At the bottom, shift your weight to the balls of your feet, swing your arms forward, and stand back up. If done properly the motion feels circular
- bootstrapper squat – stand with your feet close together, and then bend down and put your palms on the floor. Squat down onto the balls of your feet and then, keeping your hands on the floor, straighten your legs. You will feel a stretch in your hamstrings at the top. This version places much more emphasis on the quadriceps
- single-leg squat – start by standing on one leg, with your other leg tucked up under you: the leg is bent at the knee, with the hamstring flexed and the hip straight. Keep your arms outstretched in front of your body for balance. Squat down until your bent knee touches the floor; your hip will flex as you descend. When learning this move, it is helpful to touch something for balance if necessary or to squat down only part of the way until your strength improves
- pistol – this is a version of the single-leg squat. Keep your free leg and your arms extended in front of your body. Sit back, staying on your heel during the squat. This version takes a great deal of balance and strength. Start by sitting back on a chair or box and gradually lower the surface as you improve

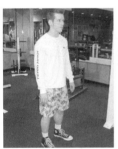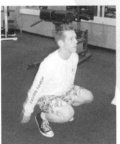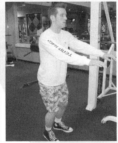

Hindu squat.

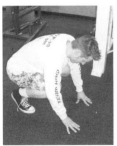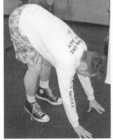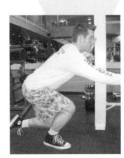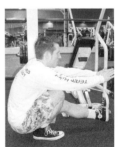

Bootstrapper squat.

Single-leg squat, bottom position.

Pistol, bottom position.

Lunges – like squats, lunges are excellent for lower-body strength and endurance. They use a lot of muscle mass and will spike your heart rate very quickly.

- stationary – step out to the front, side, or rear and step back to the start position. Repeat on the other leg
- walking – step out to the front, side, or rear, and bring the trailing leg up to meet the stepping leg so that you are moving across the floor; you can also take a long step so that the trailing leg becomes the lead leg when you put your foot down; alternate legs
- crossover – step your right leg across the front of your left leg and out to the side. Descend into a squat position and step back to the start position; repeat on the other side
- jumping lunge – lunge out and then jump up and switch leg positions, landing in a lunge on the other side

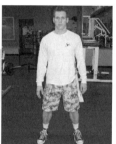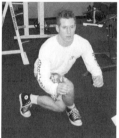

Crossover lunge.

Push-ups – this standard movement is a great conditioner for the arms, shoulders, and chest.

- hand placement – variations in hand placement can change the emphasis of the exercise. Some of these include wide or narrow spacing; fingers facing in; one arm elevated on a medicine ball; on fingertips or knuckles; or with hands on a wobble board or stability ball
- hand or foot elevation – performing push-ups with your upper body elevated on steps or a bar will make the exercises easier, while elevating the feet will make it harder
- Hindu push-up – also known as dive bombers, these place added emphasis on the shoulders and lats. Start in a push-up position with your rear in the air. Descend while moving forward, just touching your chest to the floor. Finish in an arched-back position. Reverse the movement back to the start position
- walkout push-up – begin in a standing position. Put your palms on the floor and walk out into a push-up position. Do one or more push-ups, and then walk your hands back and return to standing
- explosive push-up – descend into the push-up, and then explode up so that your hands leave the ground; these can be done with or without a clap in midair
- ring push-up – perform the push-ups on a set of gymnastic rings
- push-up step-up – get into a push-up position in front of a low box or bench. Perform step-ups by placing one hand on the box, then the other. Once both hands are on the box, step down with your hands using the opposite motion. Keep your back straight throughout the exercise. Do these for repetitions or time

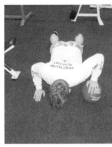

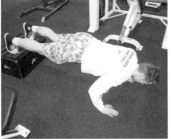

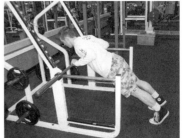

Off-set push-up, one arm elevated on medicine ball.

Push-up, feet elevated.

Push-up, hands elevated.

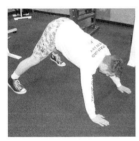

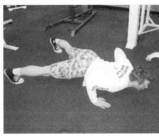

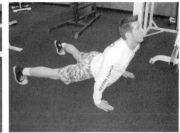

Hindu push-up.

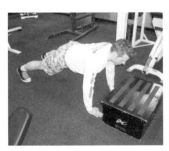

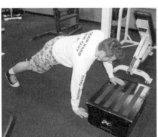

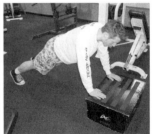

Push-up step-up.

Pull-ups – these are great for building the upper-body pulling muscles and grip strength.

- grip variations – hand placement changes the emphasis and difficulty of pull-ups. Possibilities include wide or narrow hand spacing; pronated, semi-supinated, or supinated grips; over and under (like deadlifts); or commando style
- rope/towel – to work your grip more, hang a rope or towel over the bar and grasp it for your pull-ups
- assisted/resisted – if regular pull-ups are too difficult, have a partner assist you by pushing up on your waist; conversely, use a weight vest or weighted chin–dip belt to make the pull-ups harder

- reclining pull-up – to make the exercise easier or to change the angle of the pull, perform pull-ups while lying down under a bar or Smith machine. Elevate your feet on a bench to make it more difficult
- flexed hang/slow negative – to work isometrically or to build up to a single pull-up, jump or have someone help you into the top position. Hang for a four count and then lower yourself slowly for a four count

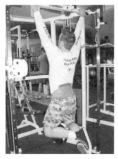 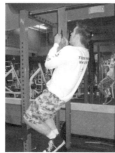 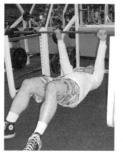 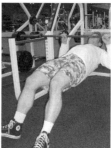

Pull-up.   Towel pull-up.   Reclining pull-up.

Dips – dips hit the shoulders, triceps, and chest. Some of the following variations may not be comfortable for some people. Find a position and range of motion that do not cause pain or overly stretch your shoulders.

- hand spacing – you can use narrower or wider hand spacing. Typically a wider hand position will allow a lower descent
- forward lean – leaning forward into the dip tends to hit the chest more; and an upright position, the triceps
- bench dip – for more triceps emphasis and to make the exercise easier, perform dips on the edge of a bench or box with your feet elevated on another bench
- ring dip – perform dips on gymnastic rings rather than bars. This version requires a lot more shoulder strength and stability

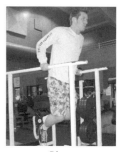

Dips.

Muscle up – this exercise is a combination of a pull-up and dip. Hang from a pair of gymnastic rings. Pull yourself up and then continue the motion, finishing with your arms locked out as in the top position of a dip. Use a spotter or slight jump to assist you until your strength improves.

Rope climbs – rope climbs are an old-school staple. Climbing ropes come in various lengths and with or without knots. The knots tend to make a rope easier to climb.

- no legs – for more upper-body emphasis, perform the climb without using your legs to help. Your legs can be held either straight down or in an L-seat position
- donkey kong – climb between two ropes, using one hand on each rope
- rope drag – if you don't have a place to hang a climbing rope, you can attach one end of a rope to a stable post and drag yourself along the floor instead. Sit on a towel or sled to reduce friction. These can be done sitting up or lying down on your back or front

Monkey bars and ladders – most people think of monkey bars as children's play equipment rather than tools for the serious athlete. If you haven't been on a set since you were a kid, a few trips back and forth will remind you of just how challenging they can be. To train with monkey bars, you can go to a park or install your own set. You can climb them in many different ways:

- forward, backward, or sideways
- walk one rung at a time or skip rungs
- explosively hop from one rung to the next
- incorporate pull-ups or hanging abdominal exercises

A ladder can be used to improvise monkey bars if you don't have a set. Angle a sturdy ladder against a wall and brace it at the bottom. Get on the inside of the ladder and climb up and down the rungs with your back facing the wall.

Crawls - crawls are a great way to work your arms and legs at the same time. They are especially good for building arm and shoulder endurance. There are two main types of crawling exercises: the bear crawl and the crab crawl. Bear crawls are done on all fours with the chest facing the floor. Stay low to the ground and move at a slow steady pace.

For the crab crawl, your chest will be facing the ceiling. Crawl on your hands and feet without letting your rear touch the ground. Either of these exercises can be performed moving forward, backward, or sideways. Learn to switch from the bear to the crab position (and vice versa) without touching anything but your hands and feet to the ground. Practice the spin move until it becomes fluid. You can even use this move as a separate exercise. Crawling is usually done for a specified distance or time interval. Increase the intensity by crawling uphill, wearing a weighted vest, or dragging a sled behind you.

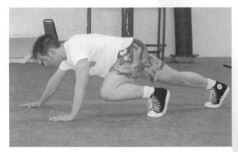

Bear crawl.

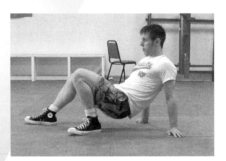

Crab crawl.

Duck walking – duck walks are really taxing to the quadriceps and calves. Squat down on your toes and put your hands behind your head. Walk forward, backward, or sideways while staying low to the ground. Keep your head and chest erect as you move. For added difficulty, these can be done up an incline or stairs. If you have knee problems, duck walking may not be suitable for you. Add distance gradually and ease up or stop if you feel pain in the joints.

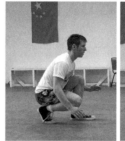 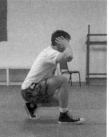

Duck walk.

Running, Swimming, Rowing, and Cardio Machines

Why would I include these after railing against them in the intro? The key is in the way they are employed. All of these "traditional" cardiovascular or aerobic modes are excellent conditioning tools; the key is not to get locked into the typical long, slow, distance (LSD) workout. LSD workout prescriptions usually follow the format of 65 to 75% heart rate max for an extended (15 to 60 minutes) period of time. Workouts like these build aerobic endurance but little else, and the endurance gains are largely confined to the mode used to train. If your main endurance training activity is running, don't expect it to transfer much to other activities, such as cycling, rowing, boxing, or grappling.

Another problem is that LSD work trains mostly slow twitch type I muscle fibers so it doesn't help much with high-intensity endurance. Sprinting recruits a lot of fast twitch type II motor units, which don't get used much during LSD training.

Using traditional cardio methods effectively to develop well-rounded conditioning requires that you vary the intensity and rotate the modality. Intensity variation involves mixing high-, medium-, and low-intensity training bouts. The trade-off is that as you lower the intensity, your total workout time will increase. Refer to the intensity zones in the section Regulating Workout Effort (Chapter 2, pp. 56–57).

The following chart will give some guidelines on how you should break down your intensity based on your primary training objectives:

Intensity guidelines

• aerobic emphasis	50% low	35% medium	15% high
• aerobic–anaerobic balance	30% low	34% medium	36% high
• anaerobic emphasis	10% low	20% medium	70% high

Note that these are not hard and fast rules, merely guidelines to help you plan your training. You could apply these over a period of 12 conditioning workouts so that for anaerobic emphasis, 3 would be low-, 3 medium-, and 6, high-intensity. Knowing this, you could then establish a rotation so that the intensity varied each time. For instance:

high – med – high – low; repeat sequence

Within each of these workouts, you can apply the interval training concept. Even on a low- or medium-intensity day, brief bouts of high-intensity work can be included. The idea is that your average heart rate falls mostly in the particular workout zone you are training.

Rotating the exercise modality is key to preventing mental staleness, avoiding overuse injuries, and promoting general endurance capability. When rotating, the heart and lungs get constant stress but the muscular requirements change. You can change your endurance modality within a workout, from workout to workout, or from week to week, depending upon your preference. Here is a partial list of possible modalities:

- running (outdoor, track, treadmill)
- cycling (with or without handles)
- elliptical cross-trainer
- rowing machine
- swimming
- walking (with weight vest and/or uphill)
- hiking
- recreational games (e.g., basketball, ultimate Frisbee)
- jumping rope

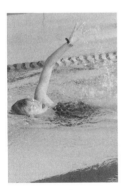

Swimming.   Treadmill.   Jumping rope.   Cycling.

Antigravity Exercise

Any exercise that requires you to support and move your bodyweight through space is considered an antigravity exercise. In essence, you must counteract the downward pull of gravity to accomplish your task. Examples are running, walking, and jumping rope. Modalities like cycling, swimming, and rowing do not require you to support and move your own weight—the apparatus or water does some of that for you. The result is that the energy demand for antigravity exercise is highly dependent on your bodyweight. It requires many more calories for a heavier person than for a lighter person to perform these activities. In the other activities, the energy output required depends on the workload. Swimming also depends on factors such as body size, technique, and drag. This is something to keep in mind when selecting modalities. If your goal is maximum calorie burning, choose mostly antigravity exercises.

An added benefit of antigravity exercise is bone loading. Exercises that force your axial skeleton (spine and pelvis) to work against gravity improve bone density. Increased bone density helps prevent osteoporosis later in life. If you are already osteoporoic or have low bone density, consult a physician to determine which exercises are recommended.

A note on running shoes

If you plan to do much running (or walking) for your conditioning, it is advisable to invest in a decent pair of running shoes. Some of the most common problems that newbie runners have are blisters, ankle pain, and shin splints, and improper footwear can contribute to all of them. If possible, go to a store that caters to runners and have them fit you with a pair of running shoes. Also, if you do a lot of running, be sure to check your shoes for excessive wear and replace them at regular intervals. Building up your endurance is painful enough without giving yourself a foot injury.

Pool Training

Swimming laps is not the only option for water-based conditioning. Water provides a very low-impact way to resist movements. Training in the pool is ideal for those who are recovering from a lower-body injury because it minimizes the joint-pounding associated with running, jumping, and other activities. You can maintain your cardiovascular fitness while your body heals so that you aren't starting from scratch. Pool workouts are also beneficial for older people, those with chronic orthopedic problems, or those who need a few weeks of active recovery from training.

- **Resisted walking**
  Get into an area that is about waist to chest deep and walk the length of the pool. Repeat for the required reps or time interval. The deeper the water, the more difficult is the exercise.

Running doesn't typically work that well because your feet won't be able to get traction on the bottom. To work your lower body in different ways, try moving forward, backward, and sideways.

- **Resisted jumping**

Jumping in the pool is similar to land-based jumping except the high impact of landing is removed. Stand in an area that is waist to chest deep and jump as high or as far as possible. The added resistance of the water increases the energy required for takeoff. You can do vertical, broad, or lateral jumps.

- **Kickboards**

Kickboards are small flotation devices used by swimmers to condition the legs while resting the arms. Place your arms on the board and hold the sides with your hands. Swim the length of the pool using only the power of your leg kick. Use a standard flutter kick, dolphin kick, or scissors kick. If you don't have a kick board, hold onto the side of the pool and swim in place.

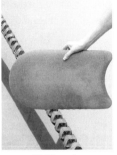
Kickboard.

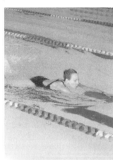
Kickboard swim.

- **Buoys**

Buoys are small flotation devices held between the thighs to keep the legs afloat, so you can swim using only the power of your arms. Swimming with the buoy is an excellent upper-body conditioner. Use a variety of strokes to hit all upper-body muscle groups.

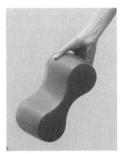
Buoy.

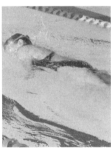
Buoy swim.

- **Poolside press-ups**

These are similar to a bench dip and work the triceps and shoulders. Place your hands on the pool side or rail. Jump slightly with your legs and lock your arms straight. Relax back to the start position and repeat for the required reps or duration.

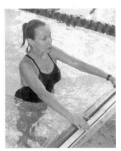
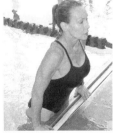
Poolside press-up.

- **Resistance exercises in the pool**

Rubber-coated weights or dumbbells, rubber bands, and rubber medicine balls can all be used while you are in the pool. Place these devices at the ends of the pool so that you can do upper-body work between laps. High-repetition dumbbell presses or other exercises can also be done while walking down the lane to increase the conditioning effect.

Exercises from Combat Sports

Due to the competitive demands of combat sports, like boxing, kickboxing, wrestling, judo, and jiu-jitsu, and other martial arts, these athletes undertake some absolutely brutal conditioning workouts. However, you don't need to actually compete in these sports to benefit from their training methods. Incorporating combat conditioning into your program is a great way to add variety.

Striking Exercises

Before using these drills, spend a little time learning how to punch and kick properly. You don't have to have perfect technique; just know how to throw your punches and kicks without damaging yourself. Learn how to jab, cross, hook, uppercut, front kick, round kick, side kick, and knee strike, and you'll know all you need for conditioning purposes. Execute your techniques from a balanced fighting stance. Center your weight over your feet to keep your balance and stay on the balls of your feet. Always keep you hands up between strikes. Not only is this a sound technical habit, but also it builds your shoulder endurance.

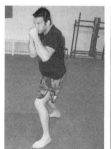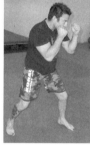

Fighting stance.

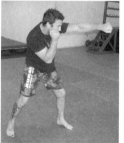

Jab.   Cross.

- **jab** – push off with your rear foot and extend your lead hand straight out. Turn your hand over so that your palm is down on impact. After you land the jab, bring your arm straight back to your chin. The other arm should stay by your head the entire time

- **cross** – push off with your rear foot and turn your hips forward as you punch straight into the target with your rear hand. Allow your feet to pivot toward the target and bend your knees slightly to get more power. Bring the hand straight back to your chin after punching. The lead hand should remain by your head during the cross

- **lead hook** – turn your arm over; pivot on your lead foot and bring your fist across to the target with the power of your trunk rotation. Keep your rear hand at your head. Immediately recover to a good fighting stance with both hands up. Punching power in the hook is generated by the torso, not the arms. Turn with your arm and body locked together as one unit

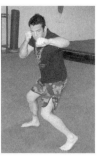

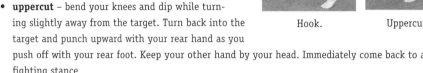

Hook.   Uppercut.

- **uppercut** – bend your knees and dip while turning slightly away from the target. Turn back into the target and punch upward with your rear hand as you push off with your rear foot. Keep your other hand by your head. Immediately come back to a fighting stance

- **front kick** – start in fighting stance. Bring your rear knee up high and then kick forward with a stomping motion. Extend your hips as you kick to generate power. Hit with the ball or the heel of the foot. You can either set the foot down in front after you kick or retract it. Retracting the foot requires a great deal more balance

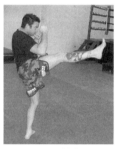

Front kick.

- **round kick** – start in a fighting stance. Bring your rear leg around, pivoting on your lead foot. Turn your hips over so that on impact, your chest is facing opposite the direction you started. Either set the foot down in front or retract it

- **side kick** – stand with your side facing the target. Cock your leg in front of you, then extend it straight out to the side. Your supporting foot should pivot so that the toes point away from the target

- **knee strike** – stand close to the target. If possible, hold on to the target or the mitt holder's head. Bring the rear leg up and drive it into the target by extending your hips and pulling with your arms. Don't let go with your hands until you complete all the reps

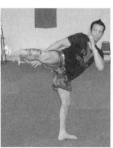

Round kick.

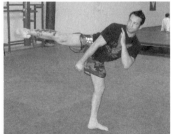

Side kick.

It is wise to invest in a decent pair of bag gloves that have wrist support to help prevent wrist sprains that can occur from a poorly executed or misplaced punch. If you want, you can also wrap your hands like a boxer. Hand-wrapping is easy to learn and the wraps are inexpensive. Hand wraps protect the knuckles and small bones of the hand from impact fractures in addition to providing wrist support. Some boxing or kickboxing trainers will insist that any trainee use wraps and heavybag gloves, while some karate instructors are just as adamant that they don't.

I believe that the amount of protection needed is directly related to how hard you punch and how much heavybag and mitt work you do. Hard hitters who use the heavybag often are at greater risk of injury and should get in the habit of hand-wrapping before workouts. If you use heavybag training only occasionally or stick mainly to punch mitts, you can usually get away without hand wraps.

Shadow boxing

Shadow boxing is throwing various strikes, kicks, and combinations as well as defensive movements in the air against an imaginary opponent. When shadow boxing, it is important to imagine that you have a real opponent in front of you. See him moving, defending, and hitting back at you. Throw a variety of techniques, putting snap into them, and practice relaxed fluid footwork. Shadow boxing can be done as a primary conditioner or as active recovery between rounds.

For boxers and other fighters, shadow boxing is typically directed toward improving a specific skill set rather than just mindless punching. This approach makes the drill more interesting and can be used to vary your conditioning routine as well.

Here are some shadow boxing workout ideas:

- perform a specific number of punches or kicks per round; more strikes in a given time make for a harder round
- perform a specific number of combinations per round; for example, 50 jab – cross – hooks
- perform specific pre-set combinations as your workout partner calls them out

Methods of increasing intensity include adding more kicks or wearing a weighted vest. Kicking uses more muscle mass than punching and as a result will elevate your heart rate more. Including an occasional squat thrust or, if you are on a softer surface, wrestling sprawl will also increase the difficulty. For more intense arm work, you can hold 0.5- or 1-lb. weights, wear light wrist weights, or use one of the rubber band systems designed for shadow boxing. The band wraps around your back to provide resistance as you punch while holding the handles. Use only light dumbbells or wrist weights to avoid hyper-extending your elbows.

Heavybag training

Heavybag training is another staple of the fighter's workout that is great for conditioning work. You can hit the bag with your best punches, kicks, knees, and other strikes and it will always come back for more. Heavybags come in various shapes and sizes. The two most common are the 70- to 100-lb. punching bag that hangs high off the floor and the longer "banana" bag used by kickboxers. The latter extends almost to the floor to accommodate knee strikes and low kicks. You can leave the bag hanging free or use a floor tie to keep it in place. An unanchored bag is preferred for developing the footwork and accuracy required to hit it as it swings, while an anchored bag is better for power training and rapid striking. It is especially important to wrap your hands or use a glove with some wrist support when working the heavybag. Otherwise, a misplaced or improperly thrown punch could lead to a sprain.

Perform rounds or do different combinations for a specified number of repetitions. When doing rounds, make sure you mix up the combinations, add ducking and defensive motions, and move around the bag rather than staying planted in one spot. Any good book or video on boxing or kickboxing will provide dozens of punch and kick combos.

A few standard punch and kick patterns are listed below to get you started:

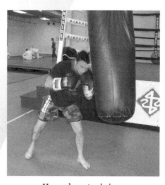

- double jab
- jab to rear leg round kick
- jab to cross
- jab to cross to lead hook
- jab to cross to straight left
- jab to cross to lead uppercut
- jab to cross to lead leg round kick
- cross to lead hook to cross
- lead uppercut to rear uppercut
- lead hook low to lead hook high to cross
- rear leg round kick to lead leg round kick

Heavybag training.

Although hitting each combo with power is the standard practice, you can build a great deal of conditioning and arm endurance by emphasizing speed. Try to hit the bag with light tapping punches as quickly as possible for a full round. To use the bag for interval work, move around it, charging in and punching continuously at full power for the work interval and jabbing lightly for the rest portion.

Focus mitts and kicking pads

Mitts and pads are similar to the heavybag except that a training partner holds them and prompts or "feeds" for specific techniques. Typically these tools are used more for speed and accuracy than for power. The small round mitts are used primarily for punching; the medium-sized rectangular Thai pads for a mixture of punching, kicking, knees, and elbows; and the thick kick shields mostly for kicks and knees. Safety is the number-one priority with mitt and pad work. Make sure you are reasonably proficient at hitting the pads before increasing the intensity, or you may accidentally hit your partner in a fatigued flurry. Pad-holding is a skill in itself. Be sure your partner knows the proper holding position for the pads so that you can both avoid injury.

The same drills performed on the heavybag can be done on the mitts and pads. Single strikes, combinations, flurries, and intervals all work well. In addition, you can incorporate movement around the room. Your partner can call out specific strikes or combos and pace you so that you push as hard as possible.

Speed bag training

Speed bags are small teardrop-shaped bags used in boxing and other striking-based martial arts. They develop hand–eye coordination and build arm and shoulder endurance. The base should be set so that the bag hangs at about your own head height. The first goal is to be able to keep the bag moving with one arm. Keep your elbow up and strike the bag with the bottom of your fist in a downward circular motion. Start by hitting the bag, letting it hit the base twice, then hitting it again.

After you've gotten the rhythm of striking the bag with one hand, begin alternating the striking hand on each rep. If you can get relatively proficient at this pattern, you know enough to use the bag for conditioning. Speed up as your skill allows. Though speed bag training may be done with bare fists, it is recommended that you wear light bag gloves in case you accidentally hit the base. If you enjoy speed bag work, you can practice further and add in many tricks, such as moving your body around as you strike and incorporating uppercuts and other strikes.

Grappling Exercises

Pummeling

Pummeling is a grip-fighting drill used by wrestlers. It develops your ability to get inside your opponent's defenses and score a takedown. Pummeling is best learned cooperatively and at a moderate pace. Once you have learned the basic movement, you can ramp up the intensity and make it competitive. Start in the over–under position: stand facing your partner with chest-to-chest contact, with your right arm under your partner's left arm and his right arm under your left arm. You and your partner swim your outside arms inside simultaneously so that the over–under position is reversed. Repeat this for the required duration. Work on smooth movement, keep your knees bent slightly, and lean into your partner for maximal chest contact.

Once you have the motion down, gradually increase the speed and start moving around the room as you pummel. Finally, turn this into a live, competitive drill. Start in the over–under position and try to get both your arms in the front body-lock position. If you get the body lock, get your hips close and try to lift your partner onto his toes. Then start over and try again.

Do pummeling for rounds, gradually increasing the time or intensity. Another option is to combine cooperative and competitive pummeling into an interval program. Go light during the rest time and fight hard during the work intervals. You'll need an interval timer or third person for this drill.

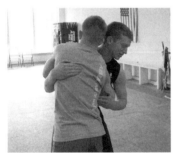 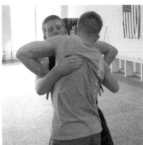 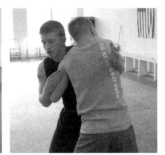

Pummeling.

Neck wrestling

Neck wrestling is a drill used by both grapplers and *Muay Thai* fighters. The goal is to build strength in the neck and lower back and learn to break the opponent's posture while maintaining yours. During the drill, keep your head up and your shoulders slightly shrugged. Maintain your balance by ensuring that your head stays over your hips and legs, with your head and chest up, one foot forward a bit, and your knees slightly bent. Your partner grabs your head with one or both hands and tries to move you around by pushing and pulling. If you lose your upright posture and get bent over, try to force your way back into an erect posture. Your partner's goal is to execute a "snap down" move by pushing you so that you must catch yourself on your hands to prevent your falling.

It is possible to make this a competitive drill with both people trying to maintain posture and force the snap down. Start with your partner putting both hands on top of your head, bending his arms and pinching his elbows together. When the round starts, try to work your hands inside so that you have both hands behind your partner's head to pull down.

Neck wrestling puts enormous stress on your neck, upper-back, and lower-back muscles as well as greatly elevating your heart rate. If you have any neck or back problems, consult a physician before doing a neck wrestling drill. Also this drill works best if you and your training partner are roughly the same size and strength. A severe mismatch can make it nearly impossible for the smaller person in a competitive situation. Be sure to warm up your neck and back thoroughly before any neck wrestling session.

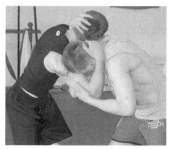

Neck wrestling.

Lifts and carries

Wrestlers and judoka frequently use their training partners as resistance implements. The two primary exercises are lifts and carries. Both build strength and endurance throughout the whole body. It is best if you and your training partner are roughly the same size and strength. If there is a difference, adjust your reps accordingly.

- **hip lift** – this move is used to train pick-up style takedowns. Squat down slightly and bear hug your partner around the waist from the front, side, or rear. Move your hips close and pop him into the air explosively, using the combined power of your legs and lower back. You must perform the hip lift with lower-body explosion and as little arm strength as possible

- **guard lift** – start on your knees, with your partner's legs wrapped around you and his hands holding on behind your head. Your arms should be under your partner's shoulders. Hop your feet forward and under you, and then stand all the way up. Keep fighting the downward pull by looking upward as you stand. A good morning can be added to the top portion of the lift for more lower-back work: after you are standing, bend forward at the waist and come back up. Avoid rounding your back by keeping your head up the whole time

- **partner carries** – carry your training partner a specified distance using one of the following holding positions: piggyback, guard, over-the-shoulder, fireman's carry, or side body lock. Carries are a great way to travel between the stations of a circuit. An alternative to the carry, if you have a suitable surface, is to drag your partner by grabbing under his armpits. Partner dragging is an excellent functional training exercise, particularly for law enforcement, military, or rescue personnel

- **partner shoves** – this exercise builds explosive driving power in the upper and lower body. Stand facing your partner with your chest almost in contact with his. Lean forward, take a step, and shove him in the chest as hard as possible. Step forward and repeat. Your partner should keep his balance so that he doesn't get knocked down. He should provide some resistance against the shove but not so much that he doesn't move. Typically this exercise is performed down the length of a floor with the partners switching roles when coming back. If space is limited, just have your partner step back to you after each rep

Sumo wrestling

Sumo wrestling is a competitive conditioning drill that is played similar to the actual sport of sumo. For safety and maximal effectiveness, you should perform this drill on a matted surface or soft grass with a partner of roughly equal size. Using tape or cones, mark out a square or circle on the floor that is at least 10′ x 10′. Make sure the area immediately outside the marked-off area is also matted and free of anything that might cause injury. Start in the middle facing your partner. The goal is to push the other person out of the ring or make him touch the mat with something other than his feet. The key is to stay low and try to get under your opponent in order to push more effectively. Another strategy is to step back sharply and pull down on your opponent's head as he pushes in order to make him stumble and catch himself with his hand. Play this drill continuously for rounds of 1 to 3 minutes, and then take a short break.

It is important that this be thought of as a conditioning drill. If you or your partner has any wrestling or judo training, you must avoid using throws and technical takedowns. The goal is not maximum efficiency in movement but maximum effort. Try to move your partner around with brute force and aggression for the greatest conditioning benefit.

Over and unders and leapfrogging

The over and under is used often by wrestlers to work on their double-leg penetration shot. Have your partner stand facing you with a wide stance. Drop low and step or dive between his legs. Your partner then bends forward as you quickly stand up, put your hands on his back, and jump over. As you touch down, your partner stands upright again and you spin around and repeat the drill. Strive to get as low as possible on the shoot-through and get height on your jump. Go as fast as possible without getting sloppy and injuring your training partner. This drill can also be done in an alternating fashion, trading reps: one person rests while the other works.

Leapfrogging is another great drill used by wrestlers and judoka as a warm-up and agility exercise. Stand behind your partner with both of you facing in the same direction. As your partner bends forward at the waist, put both hands on his lower back and leap over. Immediately set up so that your partner can do the same to you. Try to build up the pace so that you move down the floor as fast as possible.

Tire Flipping, Sled Dragging, and Other Strongman Events

Strongman competitions are a unique blend of strength and anaerobic endurance tests using numerous different functional activities. These events provide a useful source of conditioning techniques not just for strongmen, but for anyone who wants to build all-around strength and endurance. To use these exercises for conditioning purposes, find a load that will allow you to accumulate enough reps, distance, or duration to overload the heart and lungs without resulting in muscular failure.

Tire Flipping

Most of the time, worn-out tractor tires are available for free. Businesses that sell and service tires must pay to have the old ones hauled off and recycled and will gladly give them to you if you ask. Tire lifting is similar to deadlifting in that it will place great demands on your legs and lower back muscles. Start the lift by wedging your hands under the tire, driving up with your legs and back until the tire is at about shoulder height. From this position, push forward explosively with your entire body to tip it over.

Tire flips can be done for distance, reps, or time intervals. Progressions include adding distance or repetitions per set, adding time to the work interval, or increasing the number of reps you can complete in a given time. Strive to go immediately from rep to rep with little or no rest. If you have a training partner, you can alternate flips so that you get a slight rest between reps. A brief rest will enable you to do longer rounds or use a heavier tire. Tire flipping workouts also offer a change of pace from heavy squatting or deadlifting. Try substituting these for your maximal effort on your lower-body day every 4 to 6 weeks just to shock your body.

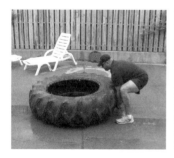 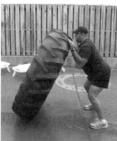 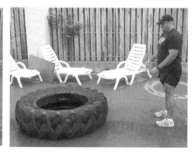

Tire flip.

Sled Dragging

Sled dragging has recently become extremely popular, particularly with powerlifters, football players, and fighters. The reasons are its versatility and its low impact on athletes whose bodies already take a beating in their sports. Dragging provides an easy way to load almost any muscle group while virtually eliminating the stressful, eccentric component responsible for delayed-onset muscle soreness. It makes an ideal modality for conditioning workouts during periods of heavy lifting or sports training and can be used effectively as a recovery workout to flush out sore muscles.

Sleds can be bought from sporting supply companies or homemade from a variety of materials. If you construct your own, make sure that it will slide without digging into the ground or tipping over. Different surfaces will provide varying amounts of traction but grass, turf, concrete, or asphalt all work well. Load the sled with weights, dumbbells, rocks, scrap metal, or anything else you have available.

- **Lower-body dragging work**

Lower-body dragging training provides the greatest overload to the heart and lungs due to the amount of muscle mass involved. The simplest method is to use a length of rope or chain to connect a sled to a weight belt or chest harness. From there you just start walking. Drag the sled forward, backward, or sideways. Change the tempo to make it harder. Long, slow walks for distances of up to a mile are great for building aerobic endurance, and shorter, faster runs really train your anaerobic capacity. Other moving exercises such as walking lunges or cariocas can be used to work other muscle groups and make the exercise more difficult. Bear crawls or crab crawls in various directions, though not strictly a lower-body move, are great for conditioning work. A final way you can bump up the intensity is to perform the drags up an incline—even a slight grade can make a serious difference.

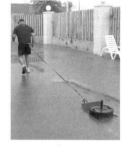
Forward sled drag.

To provide more specific overload to the hips, run a split rope and attach it to each ankle separately. Move forward, backward, or sideways, walking normally or with a stiff-legged "zombie" walk.

- **Upper-body dragging work**

The sled allows a wide variety of upper-body movements, some using a single rope and others, the split rope used in the hip exercises described above. Single-rope exercises include pulls from a variety of angles and torso rotations. To train, walk backward until there is no

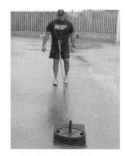
Backward sled drag.

slack in the rope and your arms are at full extension. Pull the rope to you and move the sled forward. Step back a few steps and repeat. Pull with one or two arms and at various angles. To incorporate the low back into the exercise, use a compound pull: bend forward at the waist in the start position and rise up as you pull the rope to you. Rotations are performed by standing sideways in the start position with your torso rotated as if you were in the backswing phase of hitting a baseball. With your arms extended, pull the sled using your trunk muscles.

With a split rope many more exercises are possible. For the chest, triceps, and front deltoids, you can perform horizontal presses, pectoral flyes, upright pullovers, or underhand scoops while facing away from the sled. In the start position for the drag, your arms should be in what would be considered the bottom position of these lifts if you were using dumbbells. When facing the sled you can do a variety of back, biceps, and rear deltoid exercises. Do pulls to head, neck, chest, or stomach height using an underhand or overhand grip. Perform reverse flyes for the rear delts.

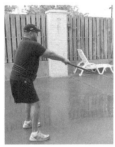 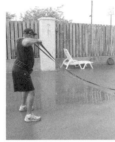 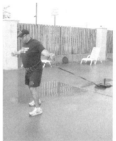 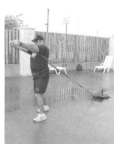

Sled drag pull with arms.   Sled drag pectoral fly.

Farmer's Walks and Wheelbarrow Pushes

Manual labor movements like these build exceptional anaerobic endurance, and grip and total-body strength. The farmer's walk is performed by lifting two heavy dumbbells and walking a specified distance. This exercise can also be done using barbells, specialized farmer's walk bars, steel suitcases, or sandbags. A low-budget method of making adjustable weights is to get two metal pails and fill them with rocks. The load will determine the distance or duration of the walk. Increase the difficulty by adding weight, distance, duration, reps, or walking uphill or upstairs.

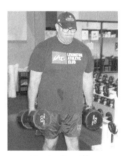

Farmer's walk.

Wheelbarrow pushes are similar to the farmer's walk but force you to work against both horizontal and vertical resistance. Load up a standard wheelbarrow with plates, rocks, or other weight and push it for a specified distance or duration. If you want a fixed weight, fill the wheelbarrow with cement and let it harden or bolt or weld weights to the inside. For an added challenge, try pushing the wheelbarrow up or down a slight grade.

Loading

Loading is another basic manual labor move that is perfect for increasing your conditioning. The concept of loading—picking up something and putting it somewhere else—is simple. When training, this can be done literally or it can be simulated with a single object. To do the literal version, you need a number of heavy objects. These can be medicine balls, sandbags, tires, logs, rocks, or anything else that is heavy and cumbersome. Start with all the items in one area, and then pick one up and move it to another location some distance away. Repeat until all the objects are at the finish location.

Since it is unreasonable to continue accumulating more heavy objects, time yourself and try to finish faster on each workout. The distance between the start and finish locations can be varied as well and will depend on how heavy your loading objects are. A loading workout can be combined with wheelbarrow training: instead of carrying the load, use the wheelbarrow to get it to the finish location. Using a wheelbarrow will allow you to do more reps in less time.

To simulate loading, you need an elevated platform and a heavy object that can be dropped without damage to it or the floor. Sandbags and no-bounce medicine balls are ideal. If you are training outside, a rock will also work. Pick up the object and place it on the platform. Next roll it off the platform and let it land before loading it again. To make the exercise more demanding, pick up the loaded object and set it back down on the ground rather than rolling it off the platform. This variation is not recommended for extremely heavy loads as it is easy to lose form and injure your back.

Car Pushing

If you've ever had the misfortune of running out of gas and had to push your car to the nearest gas station, you know what a workout this can be. And while I don't recommend you run your car dry just for the sake of a workout, pushing your car around a parking lot can get you in shape fast. The best option is to use a small car on a flat surface. Put the car in neutral and brace the steering wheel or have a training partner ride in it and keep it in a straight line. Push the car by leaning your shoulder into the trunk of the car or by putting your lower back against it. If your workout crew consists of more than two people, you can push the car in tandem with another person. You can do car pushes for time or distance. Do not ever push a car on a gradient—the car could roll back over you or roll ahead out of control.

Shoveling

Shoveling is a standard manual labor activity rather than a strongman event, but it will get you in great shape quickly. Shoveling works the back, biceps, trunk, and grip like few other exercises. If you have some landscaping or yard work to do, turn that into your workout session; otherwise, you'll need to simulate it.

To simulate shoveling, load a barbell on one end and make sure the weight is well-secured with a locking collar. If the weight is relatively light, then mimic a scooping motion, bringing the loaded end up and over your shoulder as if you were tossing the dirt behind you. With a heavier weight, this high position will most likely be impossible to attain, so keep the end lower to the ground and simulate tossing the dirt off to the side. Be sure to switch grips during your workout and train both sides of your body evenly. Shoveling can be done using a sets and reps format or continuously for timed intervals.

Indian Clubs and Sledgehammers

Indian Clubs

Indian clubs are a very ancient form of resistance training and were favored by traditional Indian wrestlers to build strength and conditioning for combat. They had a resurgence of popularity in European and American gymnasiums and military training in the 1800s and early 1900s before fading into obscurity. Today many trainees are rediscovering the benefits of club swinging due to the efforts of strength coach and martial artist Scott Sonnon.

Indian clubs are excellent for building shoulder stability and a dynamic range of motion. They also provide tremendous overload for the hands, wrists, and forearms. Traditionally Indian clubs were relatively light, but current models are available that weigh from 1 lb. up to 45 lb. It is also possible to fashion your own, using pieces of wood, tee-ball bats, old bowling pins, dumbbell handles, or other items. The weight you choose will depend on your current fitness and what types of training you plan to do with them. A variety of weights will allow the largest number of exercises.

- **Resisted leg work**

A wide variety of lower-body exercises can be done using the clubs as resistance. Perform squats, lunges, step-ups, good mornings, or other movements while holding the clubs in various positions.

Different holding positions will provide different types of upper-body isometric stress:

- shoulder rest hold
- overhead hold
- front extended hold
- side extended hold
- bent-arm front hold

- **Upper-body movements**

All of the following exercises can be performed with one or two clubs. Work slowly at first, gradually building up speed so that you can whip the club through the air and stop instantly. After you get the basic exercises, you can combine them so that each arm is doing a different movement. For a greater cardiovascular demand, perform these exercises while walking or lunging around the room. Just be sure that you have enough space so as not to hit anything or anyone. Perform Indian club exercises for sets or continuously for rounds.

- straight-arm swings – swing the club from the down position to overhead, keeping your arm and wrist extended. Swing straight up and down or at various angles across the body. Use a single- or double-handed grip

- bent-arm swings – hold the club in an upright position with your elbow at your side flexed to about 90 degrees. Bring the club up, allowing it to move behind you and then return to the start position

- circles – hold one or two clubs in the down position with your arms straight. Move the club in a large circle in front of you

- figure eights – hold a club with one or both hands and trace a figure eight pattern in front of your body. You can also do this exercise to the side or by tracing a figure eight in which one-half of the movement is in front of your body and the other half behind

- behind head rotations – hold the club like a baseball bat in front of your body. Allow it to dip behind your head, and then bring it around in a circular motion back to the front of your body

Sledgehammer Work

Sledgehammer swinging builds conditioning and work capacity as it increases grip, arm, and rotational core strength. Any athlete can benefit from gains in these areas. The first thing you need for this exercise is a sturdy sledgehammer. The exact weight will depend on your strength but for most trainees an 8- to 10-lb. hammer works best. You will also need some-thing to hit. Your best option here is a large tire. It can be the same tire that you use for tire flips or a slightly smaller one. When you hit a tire, it gives without rebounding too much. If you repeatedly hit a hard surface with a sledgehammer, the force of the impact will travel into your arms, possibly damaging your wrists, elbows, or shoulders. Lay the tire flat on the ground or angled against a wall, depending on the type of swing you are doing.

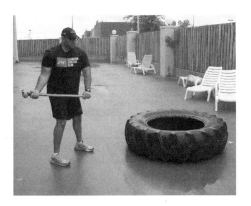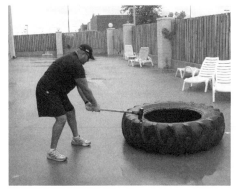

Sledgehammer chop.

- **Vertical swinging**

Holding the hammer with both hands, bring it straight up and straight down onto the tire in a downward chopping motion. The amount of knee bend you use can change the emphasis. Keep your knees mostly straight and bend more at the waist to emphasize the lower back. Squat down a bit as the hammer descends, to put more hip and gluteal work into it. Rather than straight down, you can swing the hammer in a diagonal

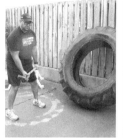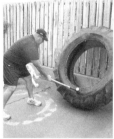

Diagonal sledgehammer chop.

motion to get more torso rotational work. Be sure to work both sides of your body.

- **Horizontal swinging**

With the tire against a wall, swing the hammer straight across your body as if you were hitting a baseball. Develop power by using your trunk muscles and pivoting on your feet. Horizontal swings can be done on the diagonal as well. Rather than coming straight across, swing the sledge downward as you pivot, striking the tire near the bottom. Repeat the motion on the other side of your body.

Kettlebells

Like Indian clubs, kettlebells were common in the 1800s and early 1900s but dropped out of sight, only to be rediscovered in the past few years. The kettlebell is similar to the dumbbell in many respects, but its unique design provides a distinctly different feel and stress on the hands, shoulders, and forearms. Kettlebells come in a variety of sizes but are usually a fixed weight. Some newer versions allow you to adjust the load. Most dumbbell exercises can be performed with kettlebells, and substituting them in your lifting routine occasionally is recommended for a change of pace.

There are some exercises though for which kettlebells are particularly well-suited:

- **Kettlebell swings**

Kettlebell swings are excellent for building power and endurance in the hips, lower back, and shoulders. They can be performed either with a single bell using two hands, a single bell using one hand, or with two bells using two hands at the same time.

Start by holding the kettlebell in front of your body, using a relaxed but secure one- or two-handed grip; the broad side of the handle is forward. Your knees should be bent, and your back straight. Explosively extend your hips and back, causing the bell to swing upward. Keep moving the bell upward until your arms are fully extended overhead. Your elbows should be straight throughout the exercise.

There are a number of different ways to perform this exercise, depending on the load and the muscles you wish to emphasize:

- swing height – to focus more on lower body work and to minimize the load on the shoulders, only swing the bell to shoulder or chest height
- continuous vs. dead stop reps – you can do your repetitions in a rhythmic motion, using the backswing of one rep to load the next one, or you can go from a dead hang on each rep
- leg, lower back, or shoulder emphasis – to emphasize the legs, squat down more on each rep. You can do extra work for the lower back by bending more at the waist on each rep. For extra shoulder emphasis, explode less with your legs and pull harder with your shoulders

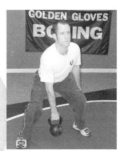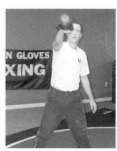

Kettlebell swings.

• Kettlebell cleans

The idea behind the kettlebell clean is similar to the barbell clean. The actual technique and feel is distinctly different due to the off-center mass. Like snatches, these can be performed with a single bell or with one in each hand. Start with the bell(s) hanging between your legs. Using an explosive hip extension and shrug, accelerate the weight upward. Catch the bells by dipping into a partial squat to absorb the shock. Some variations include:

- hang vs. pull from floor – you can perform reps from the hang position as described above or by placing the kettlebell on the floor before each rep
- alternating – when using two bells, you can clean one while holding the other in the hang position

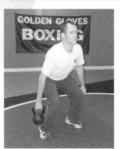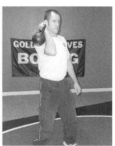

• Kettlebells snatches

Kettlebell clean.

Kettlebell snatches provide a great training stimulus for the upper back, lower back, and shoulders. They can be done with one or two kettlebells. Start in the same position as for a swing or clean. Explosively extend your hips and pull the bell as high as possible. When it reaches chest height, squat down slightly and continue to pull, catching the bell at arm's length overhead. Keep the weight as close to your body as possible during the upward pull. As you catch it, be aware that the bell will flip over to the back of your forearm. This can strain the shoulder if you don't compensate by squatting slightly and tensing your arm on impact.

Here are some ways to vary the snatch technique:

- hang vs. pull from floor – you can perform reps from the hang position as described above or by placing the kettlebell on the floor before each rep
- start position – to maximize your lower-body involvement, bend more at the waist and/or knees prior to the pull. For more of an upper-body emphasis, start the pull from a more upright position

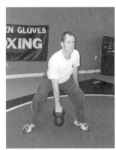 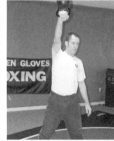 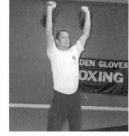

Kettlebell snatch.   Kettlebell 2-hand snatch.

- **Around the body and between the legs**

Swinging the kettlebell around your body or between your legs trains your grip, shoulders, and abdominals. For the around the body, swing a single bell across the front of your body and pass it from one hand to the other. Continue to swing the bell around and behind your back. Pass it back to your other hand and bring it around to the front. Do this in a smooth, continuous motion for the required number of reps. Be sure to do an equal number of repetitions in each direction. An excellent variation of this exercise is to switch directions on each rep.

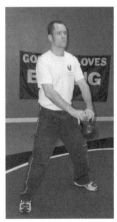 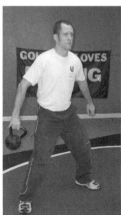 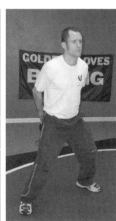 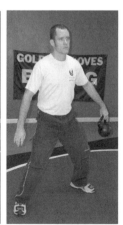

Kettlebell around the body.

Between the legs swinging is done in a figure-eight motion. Bend over at the waist and swing the bell diagonally between your legs. Pass it off to the other hand behind you and then swing it around to the front and repeat the process in the other direction. Again, set up a smooth continuous motion and do the same number of reps in both directions. Use a relatively wide stance for this exercise to avoid hitting your shins.

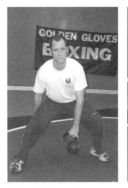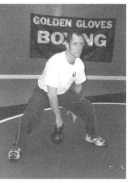

Kettlebell between the legs.

• **Kettlebell Turkish get-up**

Just like the sandbag version, this exercise works your body from head to toe. Using a kettlebell places greater demand on the shoulder than the sandbag so a much lighter weight will be necessary. Start with the bell at arm's length overhead. Go down on one knee and lie back in a fully supine position. Reverse the movement and get back up to a standing position. Your elbow should remain locked throughout the exercise. The key to performing this without dropping the bell is to keep your body under the weight. It is as much a matter of balance as strength. If you allow the load to fall to one side, you won't be able to control it and you'll miss the rep. Practice on technique is essential for this exercise.

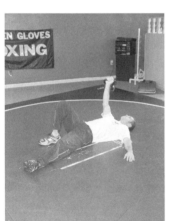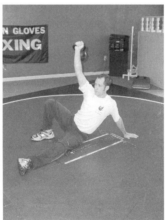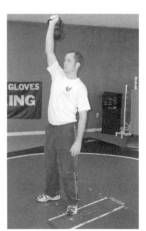

Kettlebell Turkish get-up, floor to standing.

Cable and Rubber Band Exercises

Cables and bands are nearly as versatile as free weights and can be used to train almost any movement. Cables are typically attached to a weight stack while bands can be attached to any stable anchor point. Bands come in a wide variety of strengths and most department store versions won't provide enough resistance for the average trained person. Look for bands from companies that supply equipment for lifters or athletes.

Cable and band work integrate well into all types of circuits. Although cable stacks are stationary, bands can be moved around the room to set up different circuits or can be quickly changed during the workout. One benefit of using bands for conditioning work is in the physics of the stretch resistance. When unstretched, the band has no tension. As you stretch it, the resistance increases until you reach a maximum tension during the end of the concentric phase. However, the opposite happens during the eccentric motion: as the band returns to its original length, the tension drops. The result is that you get less of an eccentric overload than with free weights or cable stacks. Less eccentric motion means less muscle breakdown and soreness—very important if you are adding conditioning work to an ongoing heavy lifting program.

Lower-body exercises

Typically lower-body exercises such as lunges and squats are loaded vertically, but with cables and bands, you can also work against horizontal resistance. Use a chest harness or weight belt to attach the cable/band to your waist or upper body. You can set up the band at the front, side, or rear and at different heights to change the direction of the pull. Step away from the anchor point until there is an appropriate degree of tension, and then perform different bodyweight or weighted exercises. Most of these are described in the section on bodyweight training:

- front, side, rear, or crossover lunges
- front, side, or rear step-ups
- squats or Hindu squats
- wrestling shots – a drill from freestyle wrestling. Perform a forward lunge, keep pushing forward until your front knee touches down, and then drag your rear leg along the floor until it is in front of you
- jumping in different directions
- walk-outs
- bear crawls
- mountain climbers

- squat thrusts or burpees
- sprint starts – starting with some tension in the band, sprint about 10 feet. Work on maximal acceleration against the resistance

If you have a continuous loop band such as the Jump Stretch flex bands, you can perform various exercises without an anchor point. Stand on the band and then loop it over your head for squats, front squats, Zercher squats, or good mornings. To adjust the tension, widen your stance so that more of the band stays on the ground.

Upper-body exercises

Cables and bands can be used for numerous push and pull exercises. They challenge the shoulder joint in multiple planes of motion and provide an excellent workout for the shoulder stabilizers. The following exercises are but a few of the many possibilities:

Presses
- high, medium, or low angles
- unilateral, bilateral, or alternating arms
- slow or explosive tempo
- step and press
- squat and press
- bend forward at waist and press
- rotational presses at various angles
- pectoral flyes

Pulls
- high, medium, or low angles
- unilateral, bilateral, or alternating arms
- slow or explosive tempo
- step back and pull
- squat and pull
- compound row with the lower back and arms
- rotational pulls
- reverse flyes
- band snatches

Core movements
- kneeling crunches
- standing crunches
- rotational standing crunches
- trunk rotations

Jumping Rope

A jump rope is one of the least expensive, most widely available, and most portable pieces of training equipment you can own. The basic model typically costs around five dollars, can be bought at any sporting goods or department store, and is easily tucked away in a gym bag. In addition to aerobic and anaerobic conditioning, jumping rope offers many other benefits, including local muscular endurance, agility, and coordination, and teaching combat athletes to be light on their feet.

Jumping rope is actually a form of low-intensity plyometrics. Plyometric training results in more efficient functioning of the neuromuscular stretch shortening cycle (SSC) and can translate into gains in lower-body explosive power. Additionally, higher amplitude jumping exercises train proper landing mechanics and may decrease the risk of ligament injury in athletes whose sports require jumping combined with quick directional change.

The standard model jump rope is usually made of rope, leather, or plastic; however, various other kinds are also available for specific training applications. Examples include:

- speed ropes – these ropes are lighter and allow the athlete to jump at a faster pace. They put greater emphasis on lower-leg endurance and lower-body coordination

- weighted ropes – available in various weights, these are typically sand-filled. They increase the overall intensity of the exercise, providing a greater upper-body workout. The trade-off is that jumping speed will be limited to some degree

- weighted handles – many ropes have weighted handles to provide more overload for the arms and shoulders during jumping; some allow the weight to be adjusted

Jump ropes can also be improvised. A length of heavy rope with some duct tape around the handles or a portion of garden hose works well. Judoka, karateka, and other martial artists also often use their belts to jump with during training sessions. Instead of buying a rope with weighted handles, wear wrist weights or hold light dumbbells.

Learning to Jump

Learning how to jump does take some practice, but it is easy to master the basic single- and double-foot jump with only a few weeks of diligent work. The key is to not get discouraged when you mess up. Start by counting the number of successful jumps before you miss one; gradually increase the number of hits from workout to workout until you are able to keep a steady rhythm for several minutes. Over time, your movements will become more efficient so that light jumping can be maintained, just like an easy jog. Unless the training activity has other requirements, relax your hands and wrists and try to minimize jump height. Hold tightly enough to maintain your grip and come off the ground just high enough to clear the rope.

The first thing you will likely notice is that your lower legs and feet will tire before your heart and lungs. By jumping 3 to 5 times per week, your calves and dorsiflexors will quickly adapt, and it will become more of a cardiovascular workout. For many people, jumping regularly is a good way to add some needed calf size.

In his book *Jump Rope Training*, former Olympic wrestler Buddy Lee outlines a three-step program to get athletes into jumping rope. He recommends building up to 10 consecutive minutes of basic jumping at a 120-rpm tempo with few or no errors before moving into more intense training. He also recommends using the basic double, single, and alternating foot jumping patterns for this initial phase before adding anything too fancy. This is sound advice. You must always crawl before you walk and walk before you run. Too much too soon will lead to overuse injuries and burnout. Those who really want to explore all the jump rope has to offer should read Lee's book.

Foot patterns and movements

At this point you can begin to incorporate some different foot patterns and movements to add variety and build agility. Each activity provides its own training stimuli and the next section covers some of the more common ones:

- double-foot jumping (DF) – jump off both feet each time. Typically the first pattern mastered by the jumper, it can also be one of the most challenging. Jumping off both feet each time does not allow any rest time for either foot, causing high levels of lower-leg fatigue other requirements

- single-foot jumping (SF) – jump on one leg. Like DF jumping, this skill is easy to master but difficult from a muscular endurance standpoint. The trained limb gets maximal over load with little rest. Be sure to train both feet

- alternating-foot jumping (AF) – jump off one foot at a time, alternating from left to right. Alternating feet builds coordination and is the best strategy for extended duration jumping. Allowing each leg to rest ensures that it does not give out before your heart and lungs

- high-knee sprinting (HK) – use an alternating-foot pattern but instead of the typical low amplitude jump, purposely bring your leg up as high as possible. Think of this movement as like sprinting in place. The high-knee jump dramatically increases the exercise intensity and anaerobic conditioning benefit

- jumping jacks (JJ) – jump first with your feet close together and then split them wide on the next jump. Repeat this continuously as if performing jumping jacks. This motion provides extra work for the hip adductors and abductors

- slalom jumps (SJ) – jump off one foot at a time in a side-to-side motion. Slaloms work the hip abductors and adductors and provide knee stability training

- bunny hops (BH) – bunny hops are two-footed jumps done with either a front-to-back or side-to-side motion, so that you are covering additional distance when jumping

- double unders (DU) – to perform a double under, jump higher than usual, tucking your knees up to your chest, and swing the rope under your feet twice for each jump. This exercise builds additional explosiveness and dramatically increases the intensity

Free Weights

In this book, free weights refers to barbells, dumbbells, kettlebells, and other weighted objects such as sandbags. Medicine balls could technically fall into this category, but because they have their own section, they will not be included here. Although typically considered tools for developing strength or hypertrophy, free weights can also be used for conditioning.

Circuit training represents the most straightforward method of conditioning with free weights. No special modifications in weight or duration must be made to your current program—just the order in which the sets are performed. For the most part, the repetitions and loads can remain the same. If you have not been doing any conditioning prior to beginning circuit work, you might have to drop back on the weights a bit due to general fatigue. However, the weight should soon climb back up as you get in better shape.

By using lower loads than those needed for hypertrophy or strength training work, free weight exercises make great total-body conditioners. Free weight conditioning circuits can be done on lifting days, following strength or hypertrophy work on off days. An added benefit of off-day free weight conditioning is that the exercises become a form of active recovery for the muscles trained on the previous day, increasing circulation to remove waste products, reduce swelling, promote faster recovery, and decrease delayed-onset muscle soreness.

Unless there is a specific need to provide additional load or to avoid loading a particular part of your body, free weight conditioning routines are best accomplished using full-body workouts. For an optimal general conditioning effect, you must keep moving through the circuit. No exercise should result in muscular failure on any set, and extreme local muscular fatigue should be avoided because it will slow down your progress through the set. The training unit is the whole circuit rather than any single exercise. It is recommended that you set up your conditioning circuits so that muscle groups are trained in a rotating fashion to provide maximal local recovery.

Choosing Exercises

While almost all resistance training exercises are suitable for conditioning circuits, the following guidelines will help you choose appropriate ones for your specific needs:

• Amount of active muscle mass

There is a direct relationship between the amount of active muscle mass in an exercise and your metabolic and cardiovascular responses. In other words, if you use compound lifts, especially those that use the legs (e.g., cleans, push presses, squats, and deadlifts), you will produce much more lactic acid, breathe harder, and jack up your heart rate more than if you did rows, bench presses, or sit-ups. Placing single-joint lifts or abdominal work between the larger lifts is one method of controlling the intensity of the circuit.

• Ease of transition

For maximum conditioning benefits you must keep moving through the circuit with little or no rest between exercises. This means that any barbells must be pre-loaded with the working weight and all the equipment used must be close by. Keep in mind the layout of the gym and move as much of the equipment you will need to one area. If you train in a commercial gym, you will also have to contend with the crowd. Plan your workouts so that you don't have to leave the weights you need unattended or you might find someone else using them when you return.

• Technical familiarity

The fatigue accumulated during conditioning work will tend to erode your lifting technique, and poor technique can easily lead to injury. To avoid this situation, make sure that you only use lifts you can do well. The middle of the circuit is not the time to get in practice reps of a brand-new exercise. If you or your partner detects technical problems during the workout, terminate the set and make adjustments for the next round. Either decrease the reps or load, or switch to an easier movement. A particular area of concern is ballistic lifting, such as the Olympic lifts and variants. These make great conditioners due to the amount of muscle mass involved; however, their high skill requirement makes them especially susceptible to fatigue-induced technical problems.

The following guidelines will help:

1. Make sure you know how to do the lifts properly and be very conservative with the load. The nature of ballistic lifts is such that very little weight is needed to get optimal conditioning benefits.

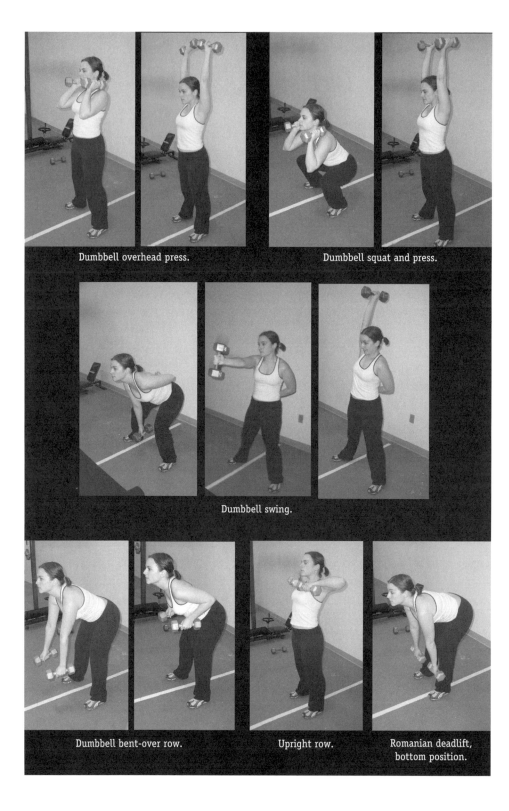

Dumbbell overhead press.   Dumbbell squat and press.

Dumbbell swing.

Dumbbell bent-over row.   Upright row.   Romanian deadlift,
                                                      bottom position.

2. Place ballistic lifts at or near the beginning of the circuit. If more than one is used in a given circuit, place less intense exercises between them to allow for slight recovery.

3. High-rep sets performed with no rest tend to cause progressive deterioration because you will not have a chance to reset your stance properly. Pause for a few seconds between reps to reset your beginning position and concentrate fully on the upcoming movement. Think of the set as a series of singles rather than one long set.

4. Dumbbell and kettlebell ballistic lifts, particularly the single-arm variations, are typically more forgiving than barbell lifts. Consider using them when your reps exceed 8 or so.

Barbell and dumbbell complexes

Barbell and dumbbell (and kettlebell) complexes have recently been popularized by such coaches as Istvan Javorek and Juan Carlos Santana. They are circuits of exercises all performed using the same weight. You run through the entire sequence without ever putting the barbell or dumbbell down. They have the advantage of reducing transition time between exercises to an absolute minimum. Complexes can be set up two different ways:

- sequenced – all repetitions of a given movement are completed before moving on to the next exercise. For example:

  Romanian deadlifts x 6, upright row x 6, power snatch x 6, overhead press x 6, squat x 6; rest and repeat

- hybrid – a single repetition of each exercise is performed before changing to the next one. For example:

  Romanian deadlift x 1, upright row x 1, power snatch x 1, overhead press x 1, squat x 1; repeat five more times then rest

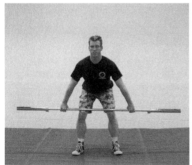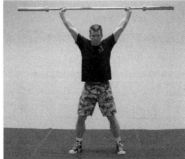

Snatch.

In both examples, you perform the same number of total reps for each exercise in a given circuit. The sequenced format typically takes less time to complete due to fewer transitions but necessitates a lighter load due to local fatigue. When designing complexes keep the following ideas in mind:

1. The load will be determined by the weakest lift in the sequence.

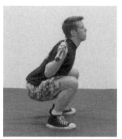
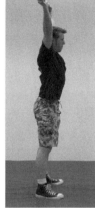

2. Your forearms and grip will be taxed heavily. Expect major forearm fatigue and place any grip-dependent exercises near the beginning of the sequence.

3. Unless you intend to emphasize a specific area of the body, rotate and balance pushing, lower-body, and pulling motions within the complex.

Barbell squat and press.

4. To minimize transition time, sequence the exercises so that the ending position of one is the start, or close to the start, position of the next. The same is true of grips used. With this in mind, review the sequenced and hybrid examples above.

Workload and progression

When using free weights for conditioning, only minor increases should be made to the training load. Remember that your purpose is to build endurance capacity, not to promote strength and hypertrophy—your heavy-lift days will take care of that. Adding too much weight can quickly shift the emphasis of the program and possibly lead to overtraining if these circuits are done in conjunction with a regular strength program. Never push to failure on any exercise when conditioning with free weights. With the training load constant (or relatively so), the main methods of progression include:

• increasing the duration of the workout by adding sets/reps
• decreasing the duration of the workout by shortening rest intervals
• increasing the density: adding more work and taking less rest while keeping the same total workout time

Core Training

Strong, well-conditioned trunk and lower-back muscles are essential for health and athletic performance. For a complete training program, you must include ample trunk work. This can be done either on lifting days, conditioning days, or split between both. You must train your core using a combination of low and high repetitions to work both strength and endurance. High-repetition work can be done almost daily, provided the exercises are rotated; however, low-repetition work should be limited to 2 to 3 times per week to allow for optimal recovery.

Plan your core training workouts according to your goal:

strength	2–3x per week	10 or fewer reps
endurance	3–7x per week	15 or more reps

Exercises

• **Sit-ups** – This old school standard exercise is still one of the best core movements you can do. Anchoring your feet under a bench or heavy dumbbells will make the exercise easier. To increase the resistance, hold a weight on your chest or behind your head, or perform them on an incline. Never pull on your neck to get extra reps or you could injure yourself.

• **Stiff-leg sit-up** – Many fitness "experts" warn against this movement because it puts a greater emphasis on the hip flexor muscles than the abdominals. However, the hip flexors need work for maximal trunk flexion strength. When performing this exercise, keep your legs about one-and-a-half times shoulder width apart. Your knees should be mostly straight, although a slight bend is okay.

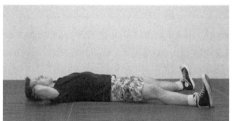 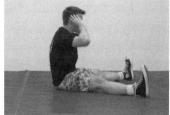

Stiff-leg sit-up.

- **Crunches** – Another basic movement, crunches are very often done incorrectly. Due to the limited range of motion you must concentrate on tension. Do this one slowly and keep your eyes focused on the ceiling during your reps. Again, pulling on the head is not recommended.

- **Stability ball crunch** – Using a ball makes the standard crunch harder by providing more range of motion. Be sure that in the "down" position, you are draped over the ball somewhat and your back is slightly arched. Cutting the eccentric portion short negates the ball's advantages.

- **Cable crunch** – Stand facing away from the cable stack with the triceps rope behind your neck. Move forward and kneel down until there is some tension on the cable. From here perform a crunch by putting your chin on your chest and moving your head toward the floor. The standing version is almost the same, except you may want to brace your legs against something to prevent being pulled backward when using heavier loads.

- **Double crunch** – Start in a supine position. Simultaneously crunch your head toward your knees as you bring your knees to your head. It isn't necessary to bring your upper body all the way off the ground. Just come up enough to tighten your abs.

- **Bicycle crunches** – Start in a supine position with your hands behind your head. Bring your left knee toward your head as you crunch up and touch it with your right elbow. Straighten your leg and relax your upper body. Next bring your right knee and left elbow together. Make sure that the opposite leg is fully extended. The exercise is good for the abdominal obliques.

- **V-up** – This demanding exercise is also known as a jackknife. Start supine with your arms extended over your head. Bring your upper and lower body off the floor at the same time and touch your hands to your feet or shins. You should fold like a book and bring most of your back off the ground. A slightly easier version involves using one leg at a time. The hardest part of this exercise is timing: your upper and lower body should go up and down at the same time.

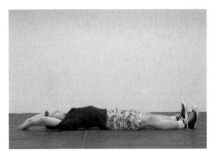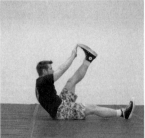

V-up.

- **Knee tuck** – Sit with your legs straight and lifted slightly off the floor, and your back at a 45-degree angle to the floor, using your hands for support. Bring both knees to your chest at the same time and then extend them back to the starting position. You can make this exercise more difficult by not using your hands for balance and support

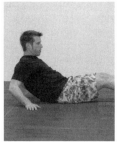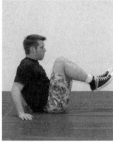

Knee tuck.

- **Hanging leg raise** – Hang from a pull-up bar and bring your legs up in front of you to a 90-degree angle. Keep your legs straight and avoid swinging. An easier version involves bending your legs and bringing up your knees. To increase the difficulty, raise your legs all the way up until your feet touch the bar. You can also do leg and knee raises on a dip stand. Support yourself with your elbows locked.

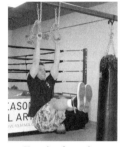

Hanging leg raise.

- **Supine leg raise** – Lie flat on your back with your hands under your lower back. Raise your legs until they are straight up in the air, and then lower them to the point just before they touch the ground. If this version is too difficult, keep your knees bent and lower your feet to the ground.

- **Flutter kick** – Sit with your body at a 45-degree angle and your legs off the floor. Brace yourself with your arms behind you. Keep your legs straight as you raise one and then the other in a swimming-kick motion.

- **Hip-ups** – Lie on your back with your legs straight up in the air. Keep your hands under your lower back. Push your feet toward the ceiling using the power of your lower abs. This exercise has a short range of motion. Try to do each rep as slowly and with as much control as possible and avoid thrusting up your legs with your hips.

- **Russian twist** – Sit on the floor in a half sit-up position with your feet anchored under a bench. Hold a medicine ball, dumbbell, or weight at arm's length from your chest. Twist side to side, using the power of your trunk. A common mistake is to move the weight side to side using only your arms—make sure to do the motion with the abdominals. You can also do this in a standing position.

- **Hip rolls** – Lie flat on your back with your arms out at your sides and your feet up in the air. Lower both legs to your right side. Let them touch the floor lightly and then reverse directions and lower them to the left side. If the straight-leg version is too difficult, keep your knees bent.

- **Torso circle** – This exercise builds strength and endurance throughout the entire core. Hold a medicine ball, dumbbell, or weight straight overhead with both hands. Moving from the waist, trace a large circle in front of you. Bend as far to the side and forward as possible to get the greatest range of motion.

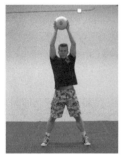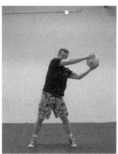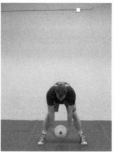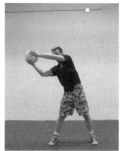

Torso circle.

- **Diagonal chop** – Hold a weight in one or both hands. Starting high on one side, bring the weight down to the low position on the other side, as if you were using an axe. Swing by using the power of your trunk rather than your arms. Pivot on the balls of your feet as you swing to allow greater range of motion and prevent knee strains. The straighter you keep your arms, the harder the exercise. Repeat on the other side.

- **Sidebend** – These build lateral trunk flexion, which many athletes sorely lack. Stand holding a dumbbell, barbell, or barbell plate at your side. Allow the weight to pull you sideways and then come back to an upright position. Be sure to keep your chest facing forward. Saxon sidebends, named for strongman Arthur Saxon, are sidebends done with a barbell held overhead in a snatch position. These will be difficult at first, so start light until you get the feel for the exercise.

- **Windmill** – Hold a dumbbell, kettlebell, or barbell overhead with one hand. Bend forward, twisting your body as you descend, until you touch the floor with the hand not holding the weight. Reverse the motion and return to the start position. The arm holding the weight remains straight throughout the exercise. Windmills are extremely difficult at first, even with a modest weight. Look up at the weight as you do each rep and keep it directly over your body. If you allow it to tip to one side, it is difficult to recover. Use only a weight that you can control.

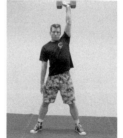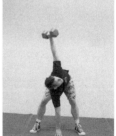

Windmill.

- **Full contact twist** – Place one end of an unloaded barbell in a corner and hold the other end at head-height with both hands. Pivot on your feet and twist side to side. Your arms should remain straight during the movement.

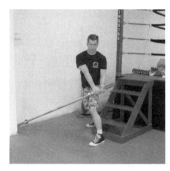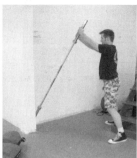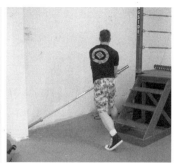

Full contact twist.

- **Superman** – The superman is a basic lower-back exercise that is appropriate for beginners and advanced athletes. Lie flat on your stomach with your arms stretched out in front of you. Simultaneously bring your arms, chest, and legs off the floor, reaching out and forward with your arms and extending back with your legs. Avoid over-arching your back. Pause for a second in the top position and then relax back to the starting position. Do not rush this one: use a slow, deliberate tempo on each rep.

- **Alternate arm/leg raise** – Start the exercise on all fours. Raise your right arm and point it straight ahead as you extend your left leg behind you. Next raise the left arm and right leg. Pause briefly at the top of the motion to keep tension on your lower back.

- **Back extension** – Use a back extension or glute–ham machine for this exercise. Place your hands behind your head or on your chest. Lower your head until your upper body is at a 90-degree angle to your lower body. Raise your upper body until it is slightly above parallel to the floor.

- **Reverse hyper** – Reverse hypers are best done on a dedicated reverse hyper apparatus but can also be done on a high box, a glute–ham machine, or a back-extension bench. Lying on your front, start with your legs hanging down at 90 degrees to your upper body. Raise them until they are parallel to the floor.

- **Good morning** – One of best exercises to train all the trunk extensors at the same time is the good morning. Place a barbell on your back as if you were going to squat. Keeping your knees unlocked but mostly straight, bend forward at the waist until your back is parallel with the floor.

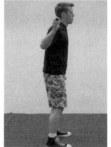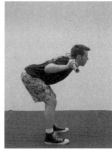

Good morning.

- **Plank hold** – Plank holds build isometric strength and endurance throughout the trunk. For the front hold, get into push-up position with only your palms, forearms, and toes on the floor. Keep your spine straight and hold the position for the required duration. Avoid letting your hips either sag or rise up high as fatigue sets in. For the side plank hold, turn to one side and get into push-up position, with only your forearm and foot on the floor; make sure that your elbow is directly under your shoulder. Keep your body in a straight line throughout the duration of the hold. Repeat on the other side.

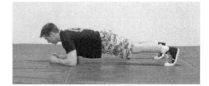

Plank hold.

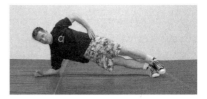

Side plank hold.

- **Overhead squat** – An assistance lift for the snatch, overhead squats thoroughly work the trunk and shoulder stabilizers. Holding the bar over head with a snatch grip, execute a full squat. The bar should be slightly behind your head. For added stability work, keep your body tight and pause for a few seconds at the bottom of the squat.

- **Sit-up and back-extension isometric hold** – You can do isometric holds with many different core exercises. For these two, just do a 10- to 20-second hold at the position of maximum tension. For sit-ups, this would be at about 45 degrees, and for back extensions, when your upper body is parallel to the floor.

For a complete core training workout, use an even mix of different types of exercises. I have found the following classification system to be useful for setting up core workouts:

Core training classification system

Trunk flexion – head to feet

- sit-ups, anchored or unanchored feet
- incline sit-ups
- stiff leg sit-ups
- crunches
- stability ball crunches
- standing or kneeling cable crunches
- double crunches
- bicycle crunches
- V-ups, single- or double-leg

Trunk flexion – feet to head

- knee tucks
- hanging leg raises (or knee raises)
- supine leg raises
- flutter kicks
- double crunches
- bicycle crunches
- V-ups, single- or double-leg
- hip-ups

Lower-back extension

- superman
- all fours arm/leg raise
- back extensions
- reverse hypers
- good mornings

Trunk stability

- plank holds
- overhead squats
- sit-up isometric holds
- back extension isometric holds

Trunk rotation/lateral flexion

- Russian twist, seated or standing
- hip rolls, knees bent or straight
- medicine ball torso circles
- medicine ball diagonal chops
- standing crunches with a twist
- sidebends
- Saxon sidebends
- DB or KB windmills
- full contact twist

Trunk training should incorporate a roughly even mixture of the exercises from each of the five groups. You could use one of each type in a single workout or spread the mixture out over a full week of training, emphasizing a different category during each training session. Trunk exercises, while demanding, do not cause so great a heart rate increase as other conditioning activities. For this reason, they can be performed during the recovery intervals from other exercises. An example of this would be:

Jump rope	3 min.
Sit-ups	1 min.
Jump rope	3 min.
Bicycle crunches	1 min.

Training Psychology

As we mentioned earlier, conditioning is not just about training the body but also the mind. Physical adaptations require forcing your body out of its comfort zone, and this is obviously not easy. It requires motivation both to begin and to continue in the face of fatigue. It requires effort, persistence, and delayed gratification. It requires that you deal with pain in the present to meet future goals. Unfortunately, these abilities are not innate; they must be developed through practice and with the help of mental techniques. By pushing yourself to your limits, you change your ideas of what your limits are. You will begin to realize that almost all limits are self-imposed. With enough time and effort you can overcome any sticking point. The following mental techniques can help you break through plateaus and take your strength and conditioning to new heights.

Pre-performance ritual

A ritual is an action that you perform consistently before or during each workout. It makes you think about training and puts you in the proper mindset to work hard. Almost all elite athletes utilize rituals before or during training and competition. The goal is a change in out-look and consciousness.

Often athletes have a different personality during training or at game time. Thoughts of everyday life are gone and the only thing that matters is finishing a set or beating their opponents. They enter a state that psychologist Mihaly Csikszentmihalyi calls "flow," where the focus is on the action of the present and time seems to slow down, and it is as if they are responding automatically to the demands of the game. Rather than waiting and hoping for this game-time personality and optimal arousal state to happen, you can anchor it to a ritual and turn it on whenever you need to. Rituals can be anything, but some common ones include:

- wearing a particular piece of clothing, such as a shirt or pair of shoes
- watching particular scenes from a motivational TV show or movie
- reading or repeating motivational quotes
- going through a particular warm-up exercise sequence
- writing performance goals on your skin with a marker

Whatever you do exclusively and consistently before workouts and competition can come to establish a particular mental state. If you have been training for a long time, you most likely have already developed some rituals. Become more aware of what you are doing, refine it, and make it more deliberate.

Attention and focus

Loss of motivation during a workout can occur when the pain of fatigue sets in and you suddenly realize how much longer you have to go before you finish. You start thinking of all the reps that lie between you and the end. All of these thoughts go on in your mind as you attempt to complete the set you're on. The result is that the workout suddenly seems to have grown in size. In your mind it has expanded into a looming monster that extends endlessly in all directions.

The key to avoiding feeling overwhelmed is to bring your attention back into the moment. Think about the set and rep you are on and nothing else. Focus only on the rep you are completing at the moment. Not only will the workout not seem so massive, but also your effort and technique will improve.

Another method of keeping your attention focused during your workouts is to incorporate meditation into your daily program. A technique known as "mindfulness meditation" will help you keep your wandering mind in check and focus on only the sensations of the present. Find a quiet, comfortable spot where you will not be disturbed. Close your eyes and focus on your breathing. Focus only on the blankness in front of your eyes. Soon you will notice that random thoughts and conversations will start to flood your mind. Notice them but try not to let your mind wander off into a long stream of thought. If it does, just relax and re-center. Start with 5 minutes or so and gradually build up your time. At first this will be very difficult, but with practice there will be fewer intruding thoughts. Daily practice with mindfulness meditation will increase your ability to attend to the present in your workouts. It is also a relaxing stress-reliever that will aid in your recovery.

Creative visualization

Confidence in your abilities and the belief that you can accomplish the task you are about to complete are essential for success. It is true that belief cannot make up for a lack of physical attributes; however, it is also true that assuming you will fail is a self-fulfilling prophesy. Creative visualization involves training to see yourself succeeding in a task before you perform it. With practice, this technique can really boost your workout or competition performance. To get started, all you need to do is close your eyes and imagine blasting through the reps. Try to bring in as many senses as you can during your visualization. Imagine the sensation of your body moving and the pain of fatigue. Hear the banging of the bar on the floor or the sound of your footsteps. Your images may not be very vivid at first, but with daily practice they will become more realistic and effective.

Visualization training can be done on off-days as preparation for your next workout session or competition. It only takes 5 or 10 minutes. You can also do it between sets during a workout.

Another type of visualization involves imagining yourself in a competition situation during your conditioning work. Motivation is almost always higher during a meet, game, or match when victory or defeat is on the line. When you need to get through the last bit of your workout, think about holding out just a little longer so that you can outlast your opponents. Use a final burst of energy to score the game-winning goal or knockout punch in your mind.

Environmental Factors

Whether you work out indoors or outside, heat, cold, and humidity can play major roles in your performance and safety. Each of these factors can influence your body at rest and in response to exercise. Every year several athletes die from hyperthermia due to excessively intense workouts in the heat and humidity. However, most of these deaths could be prevented if coaches and athletes were more educated about proper training practices.

Exercise in heat and humidity

Much of the energy your body frees from the metabolism of fats, carbohydrates, and proteins is lost as heat. This heat must be dissipated to keep the core temperature from getting too high. There are four main methods of losing heat and most are affected by environmental conditions.

Radiation – Heat can be lost or gained in the form of electromagnetic waves. Indoors, radiation usually helps cool your body. Exercising outdoors in the sun is a different matter. Exposed skin absorbs almost all of the sun's radiant heat, making it harder to cool effectively. When training outdoors in the sun, be sure to wear breathable, light-colored clothing to help deflect the sun's rays.

Conduction – Conduction is the transfer of heat from your body to another solid object such as a cold metal chair. This is typically not a very important factor in cooling during exercise.

Convection – The transfer of heat from your body to air or water surrounding it is known as convection. At room temperature this accounts for about 10 to 12% of total heat loss. It is also the major form of heat loss during swimming. When it is windy, more heat can be dissipated in this way: as the air around your body is warmed, it is quickly blown away, resulting in wind chill.

Evaporation – Under normal, comfortable workout conditions, evaporation accounts for about a quarter of total heat loss. When core temperature rises during exercise, the hypothalamus triggers the body to sweat. Sweat remains on the skin, absorbing heat until it evaporates. The important fact about this system is that sweating does not cool you unless it evaporates. If you are training in high humidity, most of your sweat will drip off before evaporating, resulting in ineffective cooling and possible hyperthermia. If you are dehydrated, your body will sweat less, making it more likely to overheat.

If the body is unable to cool itself properly, even moderate exercise can result in hyperthermia in as little as 15 minutes. With high-intensity exercise, this can happen even more quickly. Some popular workout or respiratory drugs can intensify workout heat production. Caffeine, ephedrine, and pseudo-ephedrine can exaggerate heat load and could cause you to overheat quickly. To prevent any heat problems, be sure to adhere to the following guidelines:

• stay well-hydrated by drinking plenty of water
• wear loose-fitting and light-colored clothing during workouts in the sun
• avoid training outdoors when the sun is at its peak intensity; train earlier or later in the day, if possible
• on especially hot or humid days, reduce the training intensity and volume and take more frequent rests
• abstain from using stimulants during high-intensity conditioning workouts, particularly in warm or humid environments

Exercise in cold environments

Although not nearly as much of a problem as training in the heat, cold can present problems if you are not properly prepared. Heat production increases during work, so an environment that feels cold to begin with will become comfortable after even a few minutes of exercise. One of the major problems is with the extremities becoming numb. When you begin your workout, blood is redirected to working muscles by diverting it from visceral organs and the extremities. If your hands are not adequately protected from the cold, you may lose feeling and coordination. This could result in injury from losing control of a weight. In the case of extreme cold, frostbite could be a concern.

Another problem not frequently considered with regard to cold weather training is the need for a more extended warm-up routine. Increasing your core temperature takes more effort and time in the cold than at a comfortable temperature. This is also the case if you are coming in from the cold to train. In the winter months, take 5 to 10 extra minutes to get your body ready to train so that you can avoid pulls and strains.

CHAPTER 4

WORKOUTS

This chapter provides several ready-made workouts that you can do as is, modify, or use as templates to create your own routines. In these workouts I have made an effort to mix various modalities so you can see how they fit together.

Free Weight Circuits

Mini-circuits

These short, three-exercise circuits include a push, pull, and lower-body movement so that, directly or indirectly, they hit all the major muscle groups. Mini-circuits require very little space and are perfect for home training or working out in a crowded gym. In the latter case, move all the equipment to one area of the gym so you don't have to leave any of your workout stations unattended.

Mini-circuits can be used for strength and power, hypertrophy, or conditioning training depending on the number of repetitions and loads used. You can construct a workout with a single mini-circuit, moving through it 3 or more times consecutively without resting, or by performing it continuously for timed rounds. You can also use two or more circuits and go through each one fewer times. Progressions include:

• increasing the load
• increasing the reps per set
• increasing the number of trips through the circuit
• completing more trips in a given amount of time
• performing the circuit continuously for longer time intervals

You can use dumbbells, barbells, or kettlebells, or any mix of these training modalities. If you are working with limited equipment, such as a single fixed-weight kettlebell or pair of dumbbells, use the same load for all exercises and adjust the repetitions accordingly.

Circuit #1
overhead press
squat
bent-over row

Circuit #2
bench press
alternating front lunge
upright row

Circuit #3
curl
Romanian deadlift
incline bench press

Circuit #4
high pull
deadlift
floor press

Circuit #5
push press
side lunge
snatch

Circuit #6
power clean
step-up
dip

Circuit #7
squat and push press
2-hand swing
bent-over row

Circuit #8
1-arm snatch
deadlift
1-arm bent press

Circuit #9
Turkish get-up
pull-up
dip

Circuit #10
push-up
squat
pull-up

Circuit #11
power clean and front squat
behind neck press
snatch grip upright row

Circuit #12
alternating DB push press
stiff-leg deadlift
alternating bent-over row

Extended Circuits

These longer circuits utilize a variety of different modalities. They are grouped into full-body circuits, upper-body emphasis, and lower-body emphasis. Go through the routine 3 to 5 times with minimal rest, depending on your fitness level. Repetition guides are provided but they should be adjusted based on your training goals. Full-body routines should be done 2 to 3 times per week.

Dumbbell Circuit #1

overhead press	x 10
squat	x 10
bent-over row	x 10
sit-up	x 15
bench press	x 10
front lunge	x 10/leg
curl	x 10
back extension	x 15

Dumbbell Circuit #2

upright row	x 10
deadlift	x 15
incline bench press	x 10
hanging knee-up	x 15
floor press	x 10
side lunge	x 10/leg
bent-over row	x 10
superman	x 15

Dumbbell Circuit #3

power clean to push press	x 10
Russian twist	x 30
Romanian deadlift to snatch	x 10
V-up	x 15
floor press	x 10
gladiator row*	x 10/arm

*holding a dumbbell in each hand, get into push-up position; perform a bent-over row with one arm while supporting yourself with the other arm

Dumbbell Circuit #4

overhead press	x 10
squat	x 10
bent over row	x 10
incline bench press	x 10
front lunge	x 10
upright row	x 10
flat bench press	x 10
Romanian deadlift	x 10
curl	x 10
weighted sit-up	x 10

Barbell Circuit #1

flat bench press	x 5
incline sit-up	x 20
power clean from floor	x 5
hip roll	x 20
deadlift	x 5
neck work	x 15 (each forward, backward, left and right)

Barbell Circuit #2

squat	x 15
overhead press	x 10
high pull	x 10
crunch	x 50
superman	x 25

Barbell Circuit #3

snatch	x 5
front squat	x 5
twisting sit-up	x 20
incline bench press	x 5
power shrug	x 10

Barbell Circuit #4

bent-over row	x 10
back squat	x 10
decline bench press	x 10
high pull	x 10
snatch grip deadlift	x 10
close-grip bench press	x 10
power shrug	x 10
side lunge	x 10
triceps extension	x 10
Saxon sidebend	x 10

Extended Circuits (cont.)

Bodyweight Circuit #1

jumping jack	x 25
pull-up (pronated)	x 10 (or max reps)
squat	x 30
push-up	x 20
burpee	x 10
sit-up	x 15
seal jump	x 25
pull-up (supinated)	x 10 (or max reps)
Hindu squat	x 30
Hindu push-up	x 15
back extension	x 15

Bodyweight Circuit #2

dip	x 15 (or max reps)
walking lunges	x 30
reclining pull-up	x 15
bicycle	x 40
medicine ball push-up	x 10 w/right arm on ball, x 10 w/left
crossover lunge	x 15/leg
rope climb	2 x up & down
crunch	x 40

Multi-Modal Free Weight Circuit #1

deadlift	x 3
burpee	x 10
kettlebell push jerk	x 10
mountain climber	x 40
lat pulldown	x 10
agility ladder run	2 x 15 to 20 ft.
neck bridging	x 10 (each front, back, left and right)

Multi-Modal Free Weight Circuit #2

back squat	x 15
push-up	x 20
stability ball crunch	x 20
standing cable pull	x 15

Free Weight Complexes

The following complexes can be done sequentially or as hybrid sets. Remember that the weakest lift in the sequence will determine the weight. Keep the reps to 6 or fewer if you are using the complexes for strength or hypertrophy. Progress by doing more sets of the complex. For endurance emphasis or off-day conditioning, use more repetitions.

Holding on to a bar, a pair of dumbbells, or other weight for this long is very taxing on your forearms. It may take a week or two to build up your grip and forearm endurance to the point where they are not a limiting factor in the load or reps. An alternative is to set the weight down for 10 to 15 seconds each time you complete the complex to relax your forearms and let the blood move through them.

Barbell #1

stiff-leg deadlift	x 6
power clean	x 6
push press	x 6
back squat	x 6
bent-over row	x 6

Barbell #2

Romanian deadlift	x 6
high pull	x 6
power snatch	x 6
overhead squat	x 6
behind neck push press	x 6
curl	x 6

Barbell #3

curl	x 6
upright row	x 6
power clean	x 6
split jerk	x 6
front squat	x 6
front squat press*	x 6

*overhead press while staying in the bottom squat position

Barbell #4

high pull snatch	x 6
squat and push press	x 6
bent-over row	x 6
behind neck press	x 6
step-up	x 6/leg

Barbell #5

stiff-leg deadlift	x 6
power shrug	x 10
power snatch	x 6
Bradford press*	x 6
front lunge	x 6/leg
push press	x 6

*press from the front and bring the bar down behind your neck, then press again and bring it down in front. Don't lock out your arms—only press high enough to clear your head

Free weight complexes (cont.)

Dumbbell #1

Romanian deadlift	x 6
high pull	x 6
power snatch	x 6
push press	x 6
bent-over row	x 6

Dumbbell #2

curl	x 6
power clean	x 6
squat and press	x 6
upright row	x 6
front lunge	x 6/leg

Dumbbell #3

2-arm swing	x 6
overhead squat	x 6
step-up and press	x 6/leg
stiff-leg deadlift and curl	x 6
squat to press	x 6

Dumbbell #4

alternating high pull	x 10
alternating uppercut	x 10
alternating squat to press	x 10
alternating bent-over row	x 10
burpee	x 6

Dumbbell #5 – 1 DB, do each exercise left and right

deadlift to high pull	x 6
power clean to push press	x 6
Turkish get-up	x 3
swing	x 6
lunge and press w/opposite arm	x 6

Extended Complex #1 – barbell

clean grip deadlift	x 6
clean grip high pull	x 6
power clean	x 6
front squat	x 6
push press	x 6
good morning	x 6
behind neck split jerk	x 6
front lunge	x 6/leg
bent-over row	x 6
power shrug	x 6

Extended Complex #2 – dumbbell

bent-over row	x 6
squat	x 6
overhead press	x 6
high pull snatch	x 6
side lunge	x 6/leg
push-up	x 6
power clean	x 6
squat to press	x 6
curl	x 6
Romanian deadlift	x 6

Sandbag Complex #1

shouldering	x 3/side
bear hug squat	x 6
floor press	x 10
Turkish get-up	x 3/side
push press	x 6

Sandbag Complex #2

power clean	x 6
front squat to press	x 6
bent-over row	x 6
step-up	x 6/leg
drag backward	40 yd. x 1

Gassers and Line Drills

These workouts have been used for many years to condition teams for court and field sports. It is usually easy to get access to a basketball court or football field. If you can't, any field or level surface roughly equal to that size can be used. Use orange marker cones in place of the lines. Before using any field, make sure it is free of holes and rocks so that you don't sprain an ankle. It is also not advisable to do field work on wet grass for the same reason. For more traction outdoors, cleats are an option.

Gassers

Gassers are two runs the length of the court and back. If you are using a football field, run the width rather than the length. Sprint as hard as you can and change directions at the end as quickly as possible. You must touch the line with your hand at each end. Run the gassers with a specific rest interval between. Start with 45-second rests and gradually shave off rest time over the course of several weeks.

Line drills

Similar to gassers, line drills require rapid direction change and acceleration. Start at one end of the court. Run to the near free throw line, touch it, and run back. Run to the half-court line, touch it, and run back. Run to the far free throw line, touch it, and run back. Run to the end of the court, touch it, and run back. All of this counts as a single rep. The goal is to complete the run in as little time as possible. Obviously if you use the length of a football field, the drill becomes much longer and slower, with a greater aerobic component. Use the 20-, 50-, and 20-yard lines for the field version.

Add-ins

To make either of these workouts more difficult, you can incorporate calisthenics or other exercises at the stopping points. You must get the reps done as fast as possible and get back on the move. Good add-in exercises include burpees, push-ups, pull-ups, jumping squats, medicine ball throws or slams, and sandbag shoulders or cleans.

Timing and rests

Gassers and line drills should be done at maximal speed for the greatest effect. Take your time on the first run to set your pace for the day. Try to meet or beat that time on every subsequent rep regardless of how tired you are. Over the course of several runs it is likely that your time will increase. Keep your workouts at the appropriate intensity by resting just long enough between runs so that your time does not go above 25% of its original amount: if your first run is 30 seconds, your goal is 30 seconds or less on each subsequent run. If your time ever goes above 37.5 seconds (over 25% increase), you should terminate the workout. Increase the length of your rest intervals the next time.

Begin your training using a work-to-rest ratio of about 1:2 or 1:3. Take two or three times as long to rest as you did to run. Gradually scale this back until you get to a work-to-rest ratio of 1:1 or less. Keep the quality of your reps high by following the 25% rule described above. Use an active recovery rest for these high-intensity runs: walk around and focus on controlling your breathing.

Jump Rope Routines

Long, slow, distance training

Build up gradually so that you can jump rope continuously for 15 minutes or more at a low to moderate pace. Use primarily an alternating foot jump so that one foot rests while the other works. When building up, take short 15- to 20-second breaks if your lower legs begin to tire. These brief respites will allow the leg muscles to rest without giving too much of a break to your heart and lungs. Once you have built up to 15 continuous minutes of jumping, begin adding in different jumping patterns to build agility and keep the sessions from becoming boring. For example, at a pace of 120 rpm, you could repeat the following sequence 15 times:

- double foot jump   x 20
- alternating foot jump   x 20
- single foot jump – left   x 10
- single foot jump – right   x 10
- slalom jump   x 20
- double foot front to back   x 20
- jumping jack   x 20

To vary the intensity while maintaining the same speed, alternate more demanding jumping patterns with easier ones. In the following example, the high-knee sprints and double unders require a lot of energy while the alternating foot jumps allow for some rest:

- alternating foot jump   x 50
- high-knee sprint   x 10
- alternating foot jump   x 50
- double under   x 10

Pyramid Workouts

In conditioning, pyramiding refers to choosing an exercise and a maximum amount of reps, and then performing a set for each value up to, and down from, that maximum number. For instance, if you did a pyramid set of 10, you would do a set of 1, a set of 2, and so on up to a top set of 10. Then you would go back down with sets of 9, 8, 7, and so on. This scheme is the basic idea, but there are a number of ways to implement it.

The first consideration is exercise choice. With pyramids, it is usually best to pick a whole-body exercise or one that hits a lot of muscle mass. Good examples are burpees, clean and presses, or sandbag shouldering. It is possible to run two or more equal-value pyramids at once and rotate the exercises in circuit fashion.

The next consideration is the recovery between the sets. If you are performing the circuits standing in place, use a clock or timer and take 10 to 20 seconds between sets. If you have a training partner, you can use the "I go, you go" method and rest while your training partner performs his set. This option has the benefit of automatically giving you longer rest periods to compensate for longer work intervals. You can also use walking or jogging a certain distance as recovery. If you have access to a basketball court or other large area, perform a set, and then walk, jog, or run to the other end and do the next set. If you need more recovery, use an up-and-back run; if you need less, go only halfway.

Progress on pyramid workouts by raising the top value and thereby adding more work, or by cutting back on the time to complete the pyramid.

Burpee pyramids

1. Start with two pyramids up to five (1 – 5 – 1) with a 90-second break between them.
2. Build up gradually by adding one more value to the top of the pyramid every week until you can get to 10 on each one.
3. The following week do 1 – 11 – 1 then 1 – 9 – 1. Continue taking one from the second set and adding it to the first set each week until you get to 1 – 20 – 1.
4. From there, try to gradually decrease the time.

Double and triple pyramids

- burpee, DB high pull snatch
- BB squat and press, upright row
- jumping jack, mountain climber (10 – 50 – 10 by 10s)
- dip, pull-up, squat thrust
- vertical jump, MB push throw, sandbag power clean

In-between exercises

Instead of simply walking or jogging down the floor to the next set, you can incorporate moving exercises. Use an exercise that allows the specific muscles used in the pyramid exercise to rest, but that maintains a high level of general fatigue:

- agility run – high knees, carioca step, glute kick, slide shuffle
- agility ladder run
- walking lunge
- sled or sandbag dragging
- farmer's walk
- sandbag carry
- partner carry
- bear crawl, crab crawl, or tumbling

Basic 12-Week Interval Training Progression

The following interval progression assumes that you have been doing little or no conditioning work. You can easily integrate this into an ongoing lifting program by doing your conditioning on your off days and easy days. When the frequency increases to 5 days per week, put the conditioning workouts after your lifting, either immediately after or later in the day. Whenever possible, put a day between your conditioning routines, or alternate more intense sessions with less intense ones.

The intensity rating refers to the workout as a whole. A medium intensity means that the average intensity of the session is medium. Use a mix of high-, medium-, and low-intensity bouts within each workout.

The exercise mode is up to you. Ideally, choose several and mix them within and between workouts. Good choices are running, jumping rope, rowing, cycling, and calisthenics.

	Frequency	Intensity
Weeks 1–2	2 x	medium
Weeks 3–4	3 x	medium
Weeks 5–6	3 x	medium to high
Weeks 7–8	3 x	high
Weeks 9–10	4 x	3 high, 1 medium
Weeks 11–12	5 x	3 high, 1 medium, 1 low

Interval training workout breakdowns

You can divide up the total training time for an interval workout in a number of different ways. The following example shows some different ways to use 30 minutes of interval training time. They are presented in order from lowest to highest intensity. The 30 minutes does not include rest time between rounds.

1 x 30 min.

2 x 15 min.

3 x 10 min.

5 x 6 min.

6 x 5 min.

10 x 3 min.

15 x 2 min.

30 x 1 min.

In addition to breaking up the time into rounds with passive rest intervals, you can subdivide each round into high-intensity work and lower-intensity active recovery. A 5-minute round could be subdivided into shorter intervals of 15, 30, or 60 seconds. This type of training is especially good for boxers and other fighters.

The 100 Reps Routine

The 100 Reps Routine is an easy and effective way to structure a conditioning workout. The goal during your workout will be to complete 100 total reps either of a single exercise or divided among several different exercises. The heavier each exercise, the fewer the reps and, consequently, the more exercises you will use. Here are some variations:

# of exercises	reps per exercise	type of exercise
1	100 reps	full-body
2	50 reps	full-body – upper/lower
4	25 reps	push – pull – leg – full-body
5	20 reps	push – pull – leg – core – full-body
10	10 reps	even mix of upper and lower

The goal is to complete all the repetitions in the least time possible. Time yourself and beat your previous record, even if only by a few seconds, on each consecutive workout. Drop your time by decreasing the rest intervals rather than by speeding up the reps. Never sacrifice your technique to finish faster. For a single exercise, break up the reps however needed to get finished. You can complete multiple exercises sequentially, finishing all reps of each exercise before moving on, or you can do a circuit, doing a few of each exercise each time through.

Some example workouts using the template above include:

100 reps
- sandbag shoulder
- sandbag shoulder and squat
- BB power clean to push press
- tire flip
- KB swing
- KB snatch
- BB squat to press
- burpee with push-up at bottom and pull-up at top
- MB throw

50 reps
- BB clean to front squat to press – 40-yd. sled drag
- bodyweight squat – DB curl and press
- KB snatch – KB push press
- DB Turkish get-up – overhead squat

25 reps
- push press – snatch – deadlift – hanging leg raise
- handstand push-up – pull-up – 1-leg squat – incline sit-up
- bent-over row – front squat – incline bench press – good morning
- sandbag shoulder – dip – overhead squat – full contact twist

20 reps
- high pull – overhead squat – split jerk – hanging knee raise – burpee
- pull-up – deadlift – bench press – sidebend – squat to jumping press

10 reps
- incline bench press – back squat – power snatch – floor press – front squat – pull-up – close grip bench press – jumping barbell squat – curl – sandbag shoulder

Law Enforcement, Military, and Rescue Workouts

Law enforcement, military, and rescue personnel need a wide variety of physical attributes to meet any challenges that might occur in a real-world situation. They need strength, endurance, and the ability to operate under stressful conditions. These workouts incorporate exercises designed to mimic situations that people in these occupations might face.

Wounded buddy routines

This workout requires either a partner or a heavy sandbag (125 to 150 lb.). Go through the circuit 4 to 6 total times. If you are training with a partner, take turns being the wounded person. Both of you should do the exercises at each station.

Workout #1

burpee with a push-up	x 10
partner drag (under armpit grip)	x 100 ft.
partner over & under	x 10
carry partner over right shoulder (fireman carry)	x 100 ft.
heavybag punch or knee strike sprint*	x 1 min.
carry partner over left shoulder (fireman carry)	x 100 ft.
pull-up	x 5
carry partner on back (piggyback)	x 100 ft.
rear breakfall and get up as quickly as possible	x 10
sprint	x one-quarter mile

*throw alternating punches (or knee strikes) as hard and fast as possible

Workout #2

kettlebell swing	x 15
partner carry (front "baby" carry)	x 100 ft.
DB stair run (or quick step-up onto a box)	x 30
partner drag (under armpit grip)	x 100 ft.
rope climb	3 x 15–20 ft.
bear crawl forward	x 30 ft.
bear crawl backward	x 30 ft.
partner front bear hug carry	x 100 ft.
dip	x 10
duckwalk	x 50 ft.
MB slam	x 15

These could be further modified to include weapon drawing and cover moves after the exercises at each station or when moving between stations to simulate operating a weapon under combat stress. If you have more than two people, one person can call out "Cover!" at random times during the circuit. Those in the circuit must draw and cover as quickly as possible.

Obstacle course or fitness run

Obstacle courses are part of military and law enforcement training all over the world because they build confidence and the skill to advance or retreat quickly, and they get recruits in top shape. If you have the land, time, and money, you could construct your own stationary obstacle course outdoors. If this isn't an option for you, then consider installing a few key pieces of equipment in your backyard so that you can throw up an obstacle course when you're ready to train.

Take a look at this list of equipment for an obstacle course:

- pull-up bar
- dip stand
- stable hanging area for a climbing rope, gymnastics rings, and heavybag
- box or elevated platform
- set of 6 to 10 used tires

Most of these items can be made with a minimum of effort. In fact if you look around, many of the objects already in your yard or park could serve perfectly well. A swing set or sturdy low-hanging branch can be used for doing pull-ups or for hanging workout equipment. A pair of sawhorses can double as a dip stand. Your back deck or the bed of your pick-up is a perfect platform. Take note of everything in the vicinity that could be used for training.

Other useful features of your training area include:

- stairs
- hills
- basketball goals
- low walls
- monkey bars or other playground equipment

Now add in other equipment that is portable or that can be stored outside and you have an effective course that can be rearranged from workout to workout for variety:

- hurdles
- barbells, dumbbells, kettlebells, Indian clubs
- medicine balls
- stretch bands
- large rocks, logs, bricks, or concrete masonry unit (CMU) blocks
- sandbags

Many parks have a fitness trail, which is basically a running trail with exercise equipment located along the way. Usually there will be stations for pull-ups, push-ups, dips, abs, and various other exercises. The stations will even have suggested repetition ranges for different levels of fitness. These are mini-obstacle courses and are a great change of pace from training indoors, so grab your water bottle, head out to the park, and get moving. Mix up the workout by running the trail in different directions, changing the exercises or reps, and varying the speed of the run between stations.

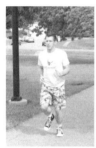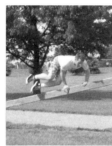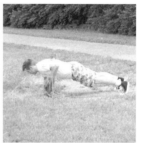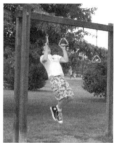

Park obstacle course.

Obstacle Course #1

over & under hurdle	6–10 hurdles
burpee with a push-up	x 5
high-knee run	10 yd.
tire flip	x 10 reps (or 15 yd.)
lateral bounding over cone	x 10
crab crawl	10 yd.
front to back bounding over cone	x 10
sprint	40 yd.
V-up	x 20
repeat	

Obstacle Course #2

Carry the sandbag with you for the entire circuit. Set it down at stations which do not use a sandbag exercise. Set up the stations about 10 yards apart.

sandbag Turkish get-up	x 6
rubber band pull	x 15
sandbag squat	x 10
MB floor slam	x 15
agility ladder run	15–20 ft.
sandbag overhead press	x 10
sit-up	x 15
vertical jump	x 10

Obstacle Course #3

rope climb	15–20 ft.
carioca step run	10 yd.
dip	x 10
bear crawl	10 yd.
jump switch lunge	x 20
jump rope run	10 yd.
pull-up	x 5
zig-zag jump moving forward	10 yd.
superman	x 20
run	40 yd.

Aqualand Circuits

Aqualand circuits combine lap swims or pool exercises and land-based exercises using the pool deck or equipment set up poolside. When arranging these circuits, you must remember that whatever equipment you use on land will get wet so you'll want it to be water resistant. Also you will likely be standing in a puddle of water, so make sure you have enough traction to perform any exercises you select. Jumping barefoot on a slippery pool deck will almost certainly lead to a trip to the emergency room.

Circuit #1

push-up	x 15
front crawl swim	2 lengths
bodyweight squat	x 25
front crawl swim	2 lengths
high band pulls	x 15
backstroke swim	2 lengths
sit-up	x 20
backstroke swim	2 lengths
superman	x 20

Circuit #2

walk in water (forward)	1 length
poolside press-up	x 15
walk in water (backward)	1 length
pull-up	x 15
walk in water (sideways)	1 length
kickboard swim	2 lengths
V-up	x 20
buoy swim	2 lengths

Circuit #3

DB squat jump and push press (in water)	x 15
rubber band pull	x 15
kickboard (flutter kick)	2 lengths
MB Russian twist (poolside)	x 20
DB squat jump and push press (in water)	x 15
DB bent-over row (poolside)	x 15
kickboard (scissor kick)	2 lengths
front crawl sprints	4 lengths

Stadium Stairs and Bleacher Runs

If you have access to a high school or college stadium, the stairs make for excellent condition-ing workouts. Try to find a run of 20 stairs if possible; otherwise use what you have available. When running up, go one step at a time or skip steps to make it more difficult. Slow the pace on your way back down so that you don't fall. Wear a weighted vest or hold some dumbbells to increase the intensity.

Workout #1
Perform this series as a circuit 3 to 5 times through with 60 to 90 seconds rest.

stair sprint	x 2 up (walk down)
all-fours crawl	x 2 up (walk down)
double-foot hop	x 1 up (walk down)
single-foot hop	x 1 up (one-half way up on each foot)
jumping jacks	x 25
Hindu push-ups	x 10
KB snatch	x 10

Workout #2

stair sprints	x 5 up (walk down)
rest 60 sec.	
double-foot hops	x 3 up (walk down)
rest 60 sec.	
single-foot hops	x 3 up, one-half way on each foot (walk down)
rest 60 sec.	
walk up and down	10 min. non-stop

Boxing and Kickboxing Routines

Boxers and kickboxers know the value of conditioning. Fatigue during a match means that they absorb a lot of punishment from their opponents. In addition they must keep their body fat level low so they can get into the lowest weight classes possible. Their workouts are an excellent mix of aerobic and anaerobic training. Even if you don't compete in these sports, their workouts can make for interesting and effective training. The only difference between kickboxing and boxing routines is technique. For boxing, you work just your hands. Kicking, however, involves much more muscle mass than punching, so if you incorporate kicks, the pace of the rounds will be a bit slower.

Routine #1

- warm-up series
- shadowboxing   3 x 2 min. (30 sec. rest)
- jump rope   3 x 2 min. (60 sec. rest)
- heavybag rounds   3 x 3 min. (60 sec. rest)
  - work single punches, basic combos, and defensive moves continuously
- shadowboxing w/1-lb. dumbbells   2 x 2 min. (60 sec. rest)
- do crunches continuously during the rest intervals

Routine #2

- warm-up series
- jog lightly and shadowbox   5 min.
- jump rope   2 x 3 min. (60 sec. rest)
- punch–kick mitt combo   2 x 3 min.; vary combos within the round
- heavybag punch interval   3 x 2 min. (60 sec. rest)
  - break each round into 30 sec. of punching lightly and 30 sec. of punching as fast and hard as possible
- speedbag   3 x 2 min. (60 sec. rest)
- do bicycle crunches continuously during the rest intervals

Routine #3

- warm-up series
- jump rope   1 x 5 min.
- jump rope   2 x 3 min. (60 sec. rest)
  - intervals: do 30 sec. easy and 30 sec. sprint for the whole round
- heavybag rounds   2 x 3 min. (30 sec. rest)
- punch mitt rounds   2 x 3 min. (30 sec. rest)
- punch–burpee pyramid   x 3 (60 sec. rest)
  - do a burpee with a push-up, then throw a single punch, do a burpee with two push-ups and throw two punches, etc. Go all the way to 8 and back down to 1

- lunge and kick   4 x 15–20 (60 sec. rest)
  - step out into a lunge position, throw an advancing front, side, or round kick then drop back into a lunge. Repeat this while moving down the floor
- shadowboxing   1 x 5 min.

Routine #4

- warm-up series
- shadowboxing   5 min.
- heavybag rounds   2 x 5 min. (60 sec. rest)
  - jog lightly around the room during the rest intervals
- heavybag sprints   5 x 1 min. (60 sec. rest)
  - punch and kick as fast and continuously as possible for the work interval and shadowbox lightly during the rests
- punch mitts   5 x 2 min. (60 sec. rest)
  - do 3 to 5 punch combinations, then immediately perform 2 burpees or tuck jumps
- speed bag   2 x 3 min. (60 sec. rest)

Martial Arts *Kata* Workouts

If you do now, or used to, practice a martial art, performing your *kata* can make a great conditioning workout. Most *kata* incorporate a wide range of strikes, blocks, and kicks to hit most major muscle groups. Choose one or more for each workout. Perform a single *kata* for the maximum number of consecutive reps in a given time. Do not sacrifice technique for speed. Increase the number of times you get through the *kata* in a single workout by decreasing the rest interval. Eventually attempt to do the reps back to back with no rest between them. If you know several *kata*, perform each one sequentially as a type of circuit. For the greatest conditioning benefit, always perform each *kata* with maximal power. Use your powers of visualization to imagine yourself in a real confrontation. This simple technique can dramatically boost the intensity of the workout. To raise the cardiovascular and strength demands, wear a weighted vest. Start with only 5 to 10 lb. and gradually build up, giving your body time to adjust to the new load, particularly if there are any jumping movements.

Heavyhands-style Workout

Heavyhands is a fitness concept developed by Dr. Leonard Schwartz in the early 1980s based on combining walking and jogging with light hand-weight exercise. The rationale behind these workouts is that you can get a better workout in less time than with walking or running alone. Performing upper-body and trunk exercises while on the move decreases your running efficiency and brings in much more muscle mass. The result is that you increase the intensity and energy cost of the workout without increasing duration or speed, providing an excellent overload stimulus for the entire body.

Walk or jog lightly for 15 to 30 minutes while performing the arm exercise patterns using a light (3- to 10-lb.) pair of dumbbells. The weight of the dumbbells should be light enough not to cause any noticeable fatigue for at least the first half of the workout. The training effect comes in the increased demand on the heart to pump blood to those muscles. Perform the sequence continuously. If you get overly fatigued, you can control the intensity by continuing to run or walk without the arm movements. Resume the upper-body work as soon as you're able. Never go to failure on any of the upper-body exercises.

Pattern #1
alternating curl	x 8
alternating overhead press	x 8
swing (ski-pole style)	x 8
chest-level air punch	x 8
shrug	x 10

Pattern #2
double curl and press	x 5
pec fly	x 5
side delt raise	x 5
twisting uppercuts	x 10

Pattern #3
outward arm circle	x 5
inward arm circle	x 5
alternating shrug (wiggle)	x 12
alternating bent-over row	x 12
alternating press out to sides	x 12

5K Build-up

This program is designed to get you from zero running capacity to a 5K distance. It is based on a gradual progression to avoid the common overuse injury of shin splints. The program is what is known as a walk–jog plan. You alternate intervals of walking at a brisk pace with light jogging, gradually increasing the amount of jogging. The program is actually based on time intervals, but you should cover roughly 3 to 3.2 miles in 30 minutes.

3 days per week (M–W–F)

- Warm up before each walk–jog

Week 1	alternate 60 sec. jogging with 90 sec. walking for 20 min.
Week 2	alternate 60 sec. jogging with 60 sec. walking for 20 min.
Week 3	alternate 90 sec. jogging with 60 sec. walking for 20 min.
Week 4	alternate 90 sec. jogging with 60 sec. walking for 25 min.
Week 5	alternate 90 sec. jogging with 60 sec. walking for 30 min.
Week 6	alternate 3 min. jogging with 60 sec. walking for 30 min.
Week 7	alternate 5 min. jogging with 60 sec. walking for 30 min.
Week 8	jog 10 min., walk 5 min., jog 10 min.
Week 9	jog 12.5 min., walk 5 min., jog 12.5 min.
Week 10	jog 15 min., walk 3 min., jog 12 min.
Week 11	jog 15 min., walk 1 min., jog 14 min.
Week 12	jog 30 min.

Core Workouts

Two-minute ab series

This drill strings together four different abdominal exercises into 2 non-stop minutes. Perform each exercise for 30 seconds, then switch immediately to the next one. Rest for 30 to 60 seconds and repeat the drill up to 5 times. Use a mix of different exercises for all-around development. To make the workouts more difficult, extend the time for each exercise by 5 seconds, add additional exercises, or go through the series more times.

Here are some example sets:

Set #1
crunch
single leg V-up
bicycle crunch
flutter kick

Set #2
sit-up
hip-up
hip roll
knee tuck

Set #3
heel touch
crunch
scissor
twisting crunch

Set #4
sit-up
leg raise
Russian twist
sit-up

Core and conditioning workouts

Good conditioning workouts can be created by combining calisthenics and other exercises with core movements. Because the core exercises use less muscle mass, they make effective active recovery for the more difficult parts of the circuit. The circuits work well following a weight training routine or on lifting off-days.

Circuit #1		Circuit #2	
jumping jack	x 25	burpee	x 10
single leg V-up	x 20	knee tuck	x 20
lateral hop over cone	x 20	jump switch lunge	x 20
hip roll	x 20	Russian twist	x 20
mountain climber	x 40	bear crawl	x 100 ft.
back extension	x 15	alternate arm/leg raise	x 20
		high-knee run in place	x 30 steps
		hanging knee-up (isometric)	x 20 sec.

Track Running Routines

Workout #1

- warm-up jog   800 m
- set 1 (shorts):
100 m sprints	x 6 (30–45 sec. rest)
200 m sprints	x 4 (45–60 sec. rest)
- set 2 (mediums):
400 m sprints	x 4 (60–90 sec. rest)
600 m sprints	x 3 (60–90 sec. rest)
- set 3 (longs):
800 m sprint	x 1
1600 m sprint	x 1

Workout #2

- warm-up jog   800 m
- set 1:
  400 m sprint repeats   x 12 (rests equal to run time)
  - if time goes above 25% of first sprint, then stop before 12 reps
- set 2:
  800 m sprint repeats   x 6 (rests equal to run time)
  - if time goes above 25% of first sprint, then stop before 12 reps

Workout #3

warm-up jog   800 m

Set up a station every 100 m for the following exercises. Run at a slow pace between stations. To increase the intensity, increase the pace of your run. Go through this circuit 4 to 8 times with no rest:

push-up burpee	x 10
KB snatch	x 10
jump switch lunge	x 20
KB push press	x 10

Workout #4

warm-up jog   800 m

sprint 200 m, jog lightly for 400 m	x 4
sprint 100 m, jog lightly for 200 m	x 6
sprint 50 m, jog lightly for 100 m	x 8

Deck of Cards Routines

These routines are based on a normal deck of 52 playing cards. In a workout, each suit represents a different exercise and the value of the card represents the reps for that set. You shuffle the deck and draw one card at a time. Do the exercises and then draw another card. The goal is to get through as many cards as quickly as possible. I read about this routine in Matt Furey's bodyweight training book *Combat Conditioning* and have used it with many different types of exercises. These routines can be used as circuit-based lifting workouts for your strength days or they can be done with lighter weights on your off-days for conditioning.

Exercises

Your selection of exercises will be based on your goal for the workout. Most of the time it is best to include one pushing, one pulling, one lower-body, and one ab exercise. If your goal is general conditioning, select four general calisthenics or three calisthenics and a core exercise. Be sure that your transition time between exercises is minimal: have all equipment loaded and nearby.

Reps

For best results, choose exercises and loads that would allow 20 consecutive reps. You can read reps off the cards with the face cards representing numbers above 10 (J-11, Q-12, K-13, A-14) or you can just call all face cards 10. Obviously the former will be a harder workout. If the reps on the cards don't work out well, as is the case with many abdominal exercises, just use a modifier. Multiply the number by 2, 3 or 5 depending on the exercise. You can modify by adding or subtracting reps as well.

Rest

Keep your rest periods to a minimum. Try to move from one card to the next with almost no rest, to the extent possible. Another option is to use the jokers as rest cards. When you draw a joker you can play it at any time to get a 1-minute rest. Try to hold onto the card without using it and only play it if absolutely necessary. If you're very fit (or masochistic), you can use the jokers to increase the intensity: when you draw a joker, you must add a positive modifier to the next five cards drawn. This modifier could be +2, 3, 4, or 5 reps, double reps, or another value that you choose.

Progressions

Progress during these routines by:

• adding weight/difficulty to the exercises
• using more difficult exercises
• going through more consecutive cards in a workout
• going through more consecutive cards before resting
• getting through more cards in a given time period
• increasing the length of your workout

Routines

- ♠ push-ups
- ♣ pull-ups
- ♥ bodyweight squats
- ♦ sit-ups

- ♠ BB squats (30% 1RM)
- ♣ BB bench presses (50% 1RM)
- ♥ reclining pull-ups
- ♦ bicycles (x 5 modifier)

- ♠ burpees
- ♣ jumping jacks (x 3 modifier)
- ♥ mountain climbers (x 5 modifier)
- ♦ tuck jumps in place

- ♠ BB squat and press (50% of press 1RM)
- ♣ BB high pulls (50% 1RM)
- ♥ back extensions (x 2 modifier)
- ♦ hanging leg raises

- ♠ 2-hand KB swings
- ♣ 2-hand KB push presses
- ♥ 2-KB high pulls
- ♦ neck bridges (do reps front, back, and both sides)

- ♠ MB slam into floor
- ♣ DB step-ups
- ♥ MB push throw into wall
- ♦ IC swings straight down to overhead (x 2 modifier)

- ♠ cycle sprints (card value x 5 = seconds)
- ♣ jump rope (card value = floor hits)
- ♥ rowing machine sprints (card value x 5 = seconds)
- ♦ sit-ups (x 3 modifier)

Other ideas

If you don't have a deck of cards on hand, use other gaming devices to decide your fate during a workout. Many games have spinners that could be labeled with various exercises. You could also make a large one relatively easily from wood and nails and hang it in your workout area. Each area can represent a number and an exercise. Spin first for the number and then a second time for the exercise. Hobby stores sell gaming dice that go from four sides all the way to 100. Make charts of exercises and roll for the exercises and reps, doing this during or even before the workout.

12-Week Beginner Strength and Conditioning Program

This 12-week program is designed for people with little or no formal training experience. It is also useful if you used to train but have taken a long time off. This beginner program uses primarily dumbbell and bodyweight exercises to correct bilateral muscle imbalances and develop body control. The goal is to raise GPP by building a combination of strength and endurance.

Use loads on each exercise whereby you are able to get all of the repetitions on each set. If you cannot complete the repetitions listed on the bodyweight exercises, adjust the resistance or lower the reps. Do not train to failure on any set in this program. For maximum benefit, complete all the workouts. If Saturday isn't possible, do the weekend workout on Sunday, or skip it altogether if you can't work out on the weekends at all.

Week 1

Monday 1

- warm-up series
- circuit A – 1 time through

- DB overhead press	x 12
- bodyweight squat	x 25
- DB bent-over row	x 12
- sit-up	x 15
- push-up	x 12
- bodyweight lunges	x 8/leg
- DB upright row	x 12
- superman	x 15

- conditioning work

- rowing machine	2 x 5 min. @ moderate pace (rest 60 sec. between)

- static stretch routine

Tuesday 1

- warm-up series
- static stretch routine

Wednesday 1

- warm-up series
- circuit B - 1 time through

- DB high pull snatch	x 12
- DB 1-arm deadlift	x 8/arm
- DB incline bench press	x 12
- Russian twist	x 20
- reclining pull-up	x 8
- DB step-up onto bench	x 8/leg
- DB floor press	x 12
- alternating arm and leg raise	x 20

- conditioning work: conditioning circuit - go through the following circuit 4 times with as little rest as possible

- jumping jack	x 25
- burpee	x 5
- mountain climber	x 30
- vertical jump	x 10
- run 100 m	x 1

- static stretch routine

Thursday 1

- warm-up series
- static stretch routine

Friday 1

- warm-up series
- circuit C - 1 time through

- bodyweight side lunge	x 8/leg
- bodyweight dip	x 10
- hanging knee raise	x 10
- seated cable row	x 12
- DB stiff-leg deadlift	x 12
- Hindu push-up	x 10
- back extension	x 15
- DB curl	x 12

- conditioning work

- track–treadmill intervals	run 60 sec., walk 60 sec. for 12 min.

Week 2

Monday 2

- warm-up series
- circuit A – 2 times through
- conditioning work

- rowing machine	3 x 5 min. @ moderate pace (60 sec. rest between)

- static stretch

Tuesday 2

- warm-up series
- static stretch

Wednesday 2

- warm-up series
- circuit B – 2 times through
- conditioning work

– conditioning circuit	5 times through with minimal rest

- static stretch

Thursday 2

- warm-up series
- static stretch

Friday 2

- warm-up series
- circuit C – 2 times through
- conditioning work

- track/treadmill intervals	run 60 sec., walk 60 sec. for 12 min.

- static stretch

Week 3

Monday 3

- warm-up series
- circuit A – 3 times through
- conditioning work

- rowing machine	3 x 6 min. @ moderate pace (60 sec. rest between)

- static stretch

Tuesday 3

- warm-up series
- static stretch

Wednesday 3

- warm-up series
- circuit B – 3 times through
- conditioning work

– conditioning circuit	6 times through with minimal rest

- static stretch

Thursday 3

- warm-up series
- static stretch

Friday 3

- warm-up series
- circuit C – 3 times through
- conditioning work

- track–treadmill intervals	run 60 sec., walk 60 sec. for 1 min.

- static stretch

Week 4

Monday 4

- warm-up series
- circuit A – 4 times through
- static stretch

Tuesday 4

- warm-up series
- conditioning work

- rowing machine	4 x 6 min. @ moderate pace (60 sec. rest between)

- static stretch

Wednesday 4

- warm-up series
- circuit B – 4 times through
- static stretch

Thursday 4

- warm-up series
- conditioning work

– conditioning circuit	4 times through with minimal rest, rest 90 sec., then 4 more times

- static stretch

Friday 4

- warm-up series
- circuit C – 4 times through
- static stretch

Saturday 4

- warm-up series
- conditioning work

- track–treadmill interval	run 60 sec., walk 60 sec. for 14 min.

- static stretch

Monday 5

- warm-up series
- circuit A2 – 3 times through

- DB push press	x 8
- jumping jack	x 20
- BB back squat	x 12
- jump rope	x 50 hits
- DB power snatch	x 12
- seal jumps	x 20
- DB bench press	x 12
- jump rope	x 50 hits
- glute ham raise	x 10
- split shuffle jumping jack	x 20
- pull-up	x 8

- static stretch

Tuesday 5

- warm-up series
- conditioning–core circuit – 5 times through, 45 sec. rest between circuits

- MB floor slam (12–20-lb. ball)	x 10
- single leg V-up	x 12
- crunch	x 20
- MB push throw at wall (12- to 20-lb. ball)	x 10
- full contact twist	x 12
- knee tuck	x 20
- agility ladder run	3 x 20 ft. (different foot pattern each time)
- rubber band good morning	x 20

- static stretch

Wednesday 5

- warm-up series
- circuit B2 – 3 times through

- DB high pull	x 8
- jumping jack	x 20
- trap bar deadlift	x 12
- jump rope	x 50 hits
- DB split jerk	x 12
- seal jump	x 20

Wednesday 5 (cont.)

- wide grip pull-up	x 8
- jump rope	x 20
- bodyweight crossover lunge	x 10/leg
- split shuffle jumping jack	x 20
- DB triceps extension	x 12
• static stretch	

Thursday 5

• warm-up series	
• conditioning work	
- burpee pyramid	1 > 8 > 1; walk or jog for 10–15 seconds between sets
- hurdle-agility circuit – 3 times through	
. over & under hurdle	2 x 8 hurdles
. lateral hop over cone (2 feet)	x 10
. front/back hop over cone (2 feet)	x 10
. forward shoulder roll	x 5/side
. cartwheel	x 5/side

Friday 5

• warm-up series	
• circuit C2 – 3 times through	
- BB step-up	x 8/leg
- jumping jack	x 20
- bodyweight dip	x 12
- jump rope	x 50 hits
- DB 1-arm swing	x 8/arm
- seal jump	x 20
- DB Romanian deadlift	x 12
- jump rope	x 50 hits
- DB decline bench press	x 10
- split shuffle jumping jack	x 20
- DB high pull to armpit	x 12
• static stretch	

Saturday 5

- warm-up series
- conditioning–core work

- treadmill walking	x 15 min.
fast walk on a 5% grade while wearing a 20–40-lb. weight vest	
- 2-minute ab drill	x 3, 60 sec. rest
. crunch	
. flutter kick	
. hip roll	
. bicycle	

- static stretch

Week 6

Monday 6

- warm-up series
- circuit A2 - 4 times through
- static stretch

Tuesday 6

- warm-up series
- conditioning–core circuit – 5 times through, 40 sec. rest between circuits

- MB floor slam (12–20-lb. ball)	x 10
- single leg V-up	x 12
- crunch	x 20
- MB push throw at wall (12–20-lb. ball)	x 10
- full contact twist	x 12
- knee tuck	x 20
- agility ladder run	3 x 20 ft. (different foot pattern each time)
- rubber band good morning	x 20

- static stretch

Wednesday 6

- warm-up series
- circuit B2 – 4 times through
- static stretch

Thursday 6

- warm-up series
- conditioning work

- burpee pyramid	1 > 9 > 1
walk or jog for 10–15 sec. between sets	
- hurdle–agility circuit – 3 times through	
. over & under hurdle	3 x 8 hurdles
. lateral hop over cone (2 feet)	x 12
. front/back hop over cone (2 feet)	x 12
. forward shoulder roll	x 6/side
. cartwheel	x 6/side

Friday 6

- warm-up series
- circuit C2 (4 times through)
- static stretch

Saturday 6

- warm-up series
- conditioning–core work

- treadmill walking	x 17 min.
fast walk on a 5% grade while wearing a 20–40-lb. weight vest	
- 2-minute ab drill	x 3, 40 sec. rest
. crunch	
. flutter kick	
. hip roll	
. bicycle	

- static stretch

Week 7

Monday 7

- warm-up series
- circuit A2 – 5 times through
- static stretch

Tuesday 7

- warm-up series
- conditioning–core circuit – 5 times through, 30 sec. rest between circuits

- MB floor slam (12–20-lb. ball)	x 10
- single leg V-up	x 12
- crunch	x 20
- MB push throw at wall (12–20-lb. ball)	x 10
- full contact twist	x 12
- knee tuck	x 20
- agility ladder run	3 x 20 ft. (different foot pattern each time)
- rubber band good morning	x 20

- static stretch

Wednesday 7

- warm-up series
- circuit B2 – 5 times through
- static stretch

Thursday 7

- warm-up series
- conditioning work

- burpee pyramid	1 > 10 > 1

walk or jog for 10–15 sec. between sets

- hurdle–agility circuit – 3 times through	
. over & under hurdle	4 x 8 hurdles
. lateral hop over cone (2 feet)	x 14
. front/back hop over cone (2 feet)	x 14
. forward shoulder roll	x 8/side
. cartwheel	x 8/side

Friday 7

- warm-up series
- circuit C2 – 5 times through
- static stretch

Saturday 7

- warm-up series
- conditioning–core work

- treadmill walking	x 20 min.

fast walk on a 5% grade while wearing a 20–40-lb. weight vest

- 2-minute ab drill	x 3, 30 sec. rest
. crunch	
. flutter kick	
. hip roll	
. bicycle	

- static stretch

Week 8

Monday 8

- warm-up series
- workout A3 – each group of four exercises is a mini-circuit; complete each mini-circuit before moving on to the next one, going through each mini-circuit 3 times

Group 1:

- pull-up (w/added weight if possible)	x 6
- burpee	x 8
- mountain climber	x 30
- incline sit-up (w/added weight if possible)	x 15

Group 2:

- single leg squat	x 8/leg
- bear crawls forward	50 ft.
- crab crawls forward	50 ft.
- hip rolls	x 20

Group 3:

- DB overhead press	x 6
- 200 m run (or run in place for 30 sec.)	x 1
- KB between legs figure 8 pass	x 6/direction
- back extension	x 15

- static stretch

Tuesday 8

- warm-up series
- conditioning work

- KB circuit – 3 times through w/no rest; use light weight	
. 1-arm swings	x 10/arm
. 1-arm clean & push press	x 8/arm
. Turkish get-up	x 6/side
- jump rope	5 x 3 min. (60 sec. break)

- static stretch

Wednesday 8

- warm-up series
- workout B3 - each of the four exercises is a mini-circuit; complete each mini-circuit before moving on to the next one, going through each mini-circuit 3 times

Group 1:	
- DB bench press	x 6
- burpee	x 8
- mountain climber	x 30
- SB crunch	x 20
Group 2:	
- BB deadlift	x 6
- bear crawl forward	50 ft.
- crab crawl forward	50 ft.
- side crunch	x 20/side
Group 3:	
- DB bent-over row	x 6
- 200 m run (or run in place for 30 sec.)	x 1
- KB between legs figure 8 pass	x 6/direction
- reverse hyper	x 15

- static stretch

Thursday 8

- warm-up series
- conditioning work

- rowing machine sprint	5 x 2 min. (30 sec. rest)
- 400 m sprint	x 6 (90 sec. walking rest)
- light jog	8 min.

- static stretch

Friday 8

- warm-up series
- workout B3 – each of the four exercises is a mini-circuit; complete each mini-circuit before moving on to the next one, going through each mini-circuit 3 times

Group 1:	
- back squat	x 6
- bear crawl forward	50 ft.
- crab crawl forward	50 ft.
- DB sidebend	x 15/side
Group 2:	
- DB incline bench press	x 6
- burpee	x 8
- mountain climber	x 30
- double crunch	x 20
Group 3:	
- DB upright row	x 6
- 200 m run (or run in place for 30 sec.)	x 1
- KB between legs figure 8 pass	x 6/direction
- good morning	x 12

- static stretch

Saturday 8

- warm-up
- conditioning work:

- circuit – 5 times through, 30 sec. rest	
. MB throw into floor (or low-angle rebounder)	x 10
. MB throw into wall (or chest-height rebounder)	x 10
. MB diagonal chop	x 10/side
. back fall	x 10
- cycling (fast with resistance)	3 x 5 min. (60 sec. rest)

- static stretch

Week 9

Monday 9

- warm-up series
- workout A3 – go through each mini-circuit 4 times
- static stretch

Tuesday 9

- warm-up series
- conditioning work
  - KB circuit – 3 times through w/no rest, use light weight

. 1-arm swing	x 12/arm
. 1-arm clean & push press	x 10/arm
. Turkish get-up	x 8/side
- jump rope	5 x 3 min. (50 sec. break)

- static stretch

Wednesday 9

- warm-up series
- workout B3 – go through each mini-circuit 4 times
- static stretch

Thursday 9

- warm-up series
- conditioning work

- rowing machine sprint	5 x 2.5 min. (30 sec. rest)
- 400 m sprint	x 7 (90 sec. walking rest)
- light jog	8 min.

- static stretch

Friday 9

- warm-up series
- workout C3 – go through each mini-circuit 4 times
- static stretch

Saturday 9

- warm-up series
  conditioning work
  - circuit – 5 times through, 30 sec. rest

. MB throw into floor (or low-angle rebounder)	x 12
. MB throw into wall (or chest-height rebounder)	x 12
. MB diagonal chop	x 12/side
. back fall	x 12
- cycling (fast with resistance)	3 x 5 min. (50 sec. rest)

- static stretch

Week 10

Monday 10

- warm-up series
- workout A3 – go through each mini-circuit 5 times
- static stretch

Tuesday 10

- warm-up series
- conditioning work

- KB circuit – 4 times through w/no rest, use light weight	
. 1-arm swing	x 12/arm
. 1-arm clean & push press	x 10/arm
. Turkish get-up	x 8/side
- jump rope	5 x 3 min. (30 sec. break)

- static stretch

Wednesday 10

- warm-up series
- workout B3 – go through each mini-circuit 5 times
- static stretch

Thursday 10

- warm-up series
- conditioning work

- rowing machine sprint	5 x 3 min. (30 sec. rest)
- 400 m sprint	x 8 (90 sec. walking rest)
- light jog	8 min.

- static stretch

Friday 10

- warm-up series
- workout C3 – go through each mini-circuit 5 times
- static stretch

. MB throw into wall (or chest-height rebounder)	x 12
. MB diagonal chop	x 12/side
. back fall	x 12

Saturday 10

- warm-up series
- conditioning work
  - circuit – 6 times through, 30 sec. rest

. MB throw into floor (or low-angle rebounder)	x 12
. MB throw into wall (or chest-height rebounder)	x 12
. MB diagonal chop	x 12/side
. back fall	x 12
- cycling (fast with resistance)	3 x 5 min. (40 sec. rest)

- static stretch

Week 11

Monday 11

- warm-up series
- circuit A4 – 5 times through

- DB squat to push press	x 8
- DB Romanian deadlift to power snatch	x 8
- push-up	x 15
- front lunge	x 10/leg
- pull-up	x 8
- DB power shrug	x 12
- DB supine triceps extension	x 12
- DB curl	x 12

- ab circuit A –3 times through

- toe touch crunch	x 20
- crossover crunch	x 20/side
- leg raise	x 20
- hip roll	x 20
- superman	x 20

- static stretch

Tuesday 11

- warm-up series
- conditioning work

- heavybag round	5 x 3 min. (60 sec. rest)

  use a variety of punches and combinations; keep moving the entire round
  - calisthenics circuit – 5 times through

Tuesday 11 (cont.)

. jumping jack	x 15
. seal jump	x 15
. bodyweight squat	x 10
. mountain climber	x 30
. bear crawl forward	x 30 ft.
. bear crawl backward	x 30 ft.
. bear crawl left	x 30 ft.
. bear crawl right	x 30 ft.

- static stretch

Wednesday 11

- warm-up series
- circuit A4 – 5 times through

- DB power clean to push press	x 8
- DB high pull to power snatch	x 8
- Hindu squat	x 30
- dip	x 12
- reclining pull-up	x 8
- DB pullover	x 12
- front delt plate raise	x 12
- DB reverse flye	x 12

- ab circuit A – 3 times through

- single leg V-up	x 20
- bicycle	x 50
- flutter kick	x 30
- MB figure eight	x 10/direction
- alternate arm/leg raise	x 20

- static stretch

Thursday 11

- warm-up series
- conditioning work

- agility ladder run	4 x 16 (rest 60 sec.)
use the following series four times for each set:	
. high knee	
. in & out left	
. in & out right	

Thursday 11 (cont.)

. 90-degree jump	
- burpee pyramid	1 > 10 > 1
jog the length of a basketball court between sets	
• static stretch	

Friday 11

• warm-up series	
• circuit A4 – 5 times through	
- DB power clean to squat to split jerk	x 8
- KB 2-hand swing	x 10
- commando pull-up	x 8
- DB jump squat	x 12
- triceps push-up	x 10
- DB muscle snatch	x 12
- DB lunge and side delt raise	x 12
- DB box jump	x 12
• ab circuit A – 3 times through	
- SB crossover crunch	x 10/side
- leg scissor	x 20
- incline sit-up	x 30
- DB windmill	x 5/side
- reverse hyper	x 15
• static stretch	

Saturday 11

• warm-up series	
• conditioning work	
- running (fast pace)	2 x 5 min. (rest 60 sec.)
- cycling (fast pace)	2 x 5 min. (rest 60 sec.)
- rowing (fast pace)	2 x 5 min. (rest 60 sec.)
- jump rope	2 x 5 min. (rest 60 sec.)
• static stretch	

Week 12

Monday 12

- warm-up series
- circuit A4 – 5 times through
- ab circuit A – 3 times through
- static stretch

Tuesday 12

- warm-up series
- conditioning work

- heavybag round	5 x 3 min. (60 sec.)

use a variety of punches and combinations; keep moving the entire round

- calisthenics circuit –5 times through

. jumping jack	x 15
. seal jump	x 15
. bodyweight squat	x 10
. mountain climber	x 30
. bear crawl forward	x 30 ft.
. bear crawl backward	x 30 ft.
. bear crawl left	x 30 ft.
. bear crawl right	x 30 ft.

- static stretch

Wednesday 12

- warm-up series
- circuit A4 – 5 times through
- ab circuit A – 3 times through
- static stretch

Thursday 12

- warm-up routine
- conditioning work

- agility ladder run	4 x 16 (rest 60 sec.)

use the following series four times for each set:

. high knee

. in & out left

. in & out right

Thursday 12 (cont.)

. 90-degree jump	
- burpee pyramid	1 > 10 > 1
jog the length of a basketball court between sets	
• static stretch	

Friday 12

- warm-up series
- circuit A4 – 5 times through
- ab circuit A – 3 times through
- static stretch

Saturday 12

- warm-up series
- conditioning work

- running (fast pace)	2 x 5 min. (rest 60 sec.)
- cycling (fast pace)	2 x 5 min. (rest 60 sec.)
- rowing (fast pace)	2 x 5 min. (rest 60 sec.)
- jump rope	2 x 5 min. (rest 60 sec.)

- static stretch

6-Week Strength & Conditioning for Intermediate to Advanced Athletes

This 6-week training program incorporates heavy lifting and high-intensity conditioning and is suitable for those who have developed a reasonable GPP training base. It utilizes a method called "complex training." In complex training, you pair a high-load lifting exercise with a plyometric or ballistic exercise that is similar biomechanically. Use the percentages given as guidelines rather than absolutes.

Week 1

Monday 1

- warm-up series
- primary circuit – 8 times through

- BB deadlift	x 3 (work up to 85% 1RM)
- jump rope	x 50 hits
- BB jump squat	x 3 (use 25–30% 1RM)
- 4-way neck work	2 x 10/each way

- auxiliary circuit – 4 times through

- BB front lunge	x 8/leg
- leg curl	x 10
- cable pull to face	x 12
- BB tricep extension	x 12

- ab circuit – 3 times through

- straight leg sit-up	x 8
- standing cable crunch	x 10
- reverse hyper	x 10

- static stretch

Tuesday 1

- warm-up series
- conditioning work

- sled drag forward	x 5 min. (moderate load)
- rest 60 sec.	
- sled drag backward	x 5 min. (moderate load)
- sledgehammer swings circuit	x 5 (60 sec. rest)
perform 10 diagonal left, 10 diagonal right, and 10 straight down on each set	
- MB throw	2 x 5 min. (60 sec. rest)
use a 20–30-lb. ball and throw it as far as you can; jog/walk to it and repeat for the entire round; use a variety of throwing techniques	

- static stretch

Wednesday 1

- warm-up series
- primary circuit – 8 times through

- incline bench press	x 3 (work up to 85% 1RM)
- jumping jack	x 30
- explosive push-up	x 3 (use about 25–30% 1RM)
- neck bridge	x 12/each way (do 2 sets in each direction)

- auxiliary circuit – 4 times through

- bodyweight dip	x 12
- DB flye	x 12
- glute ham raise	x 10
- BB reverse curl	x 12

- ab circuit – 3 times through

- hanging leg raise	x 10
- full contact twist	x 12
- back extension	x 12

- static stretch

Thursday 1

- warm-up series
- conditioning work

  - Tabata intervals - 20 sec. work: 10 sec. rest, done 8 times for each exercise; rest 60 sec. between exercises:

  burpee – DB squat to overhead press – jumping step-up – high-knee run in place

- stairway walking	x 10 min.

  wear a 20–40-lb. weight vest or hold dumbbells; a stair-stepper cardio machine or treadmill set to a 5–10 degree incline may be used if you don't have stairs

- static stretch

Friday 1

- warm-up series
- primary circuit – 8 times through

- BB bent-over row	x 3 (work up to 85% 1RM)
- jumping step-up	x 30
- DB snatch	x 3 (use about 25–30% 1RM)
- partner neck work	x 12/each way (do 2 sets in each direction)

- auxiliary circuit – 4 times through

- pull-up	x 10 (or max reps)

Friday 1 (cont.)

- BB shrug	x 10
- tricep pressdown	x 12
- side lunge	x 10/leg
• ab circuit – 3 times through	
- V-up	x 12
- DB sidebend	x 10/side
- superman	x 20
• static stretch	

Saturday 1 (optional)

- • warm-up series
- • 20 min. jog at moderate pace
- • static stretch

Week 2

Monday 2

- • warm-up series
- • primary circuit (8 times through)

- BB deadlift	x 3 (work up to 87.5% 1RM)
- jump rope	x 50 hits
- BB jump squat	x 4 (use about 25–30% 1RM)
- 4-way neck work	x 12/each way (do 2 sets in each direction)

- • auxiliary circuit – 4 times through

- BB front lunge	x 9/leg
- leg curl	x 11
- cable pull to face	x 13
- BB tricep extension	x 13

- • ab circuit – 3 times through

- straight-leg sit-up	x 9
- standing cable crunch	x 11
- reverse hyper	x 11
• static stretch	

Tuesday 2

- • warm-up series
- • conditioning work

- sled drag forward	x 5 min. (moderate load)
- rest 50 sec.	
- sled drag backward	x 5 min. (moderate load)
- sledgehammer swing circuit	x 5 (50 sec. rest)
perform 10 diagonal left, 10 diagonal right, and 10 straight down on each set	
- medicine ball throw	2 x 5 min. (50 sec. rest)
use a 20–30-lb. ball and throw it as far as you can; jog/walk to it and repeat	
for the entire round; use a variety of throwing techniques	

- static stretch

Wednesday 2

- warm-up series
- primary circuit – 8 times through

- incline bench press	x 3 (work up to 87.5% 1RM)
- jumping jack	x 30
- explosive push-up	x 4 (use about 25–30% 1RM)
- neck bridge	x 13/each way (do 2 sets in each direction)

- auxiliary circuit – 4 times through

- bodyweight dip	x 13
- DB flye	x 13
- glute ham raise	x 11
- BB reverse curl	x 13

- ab circuit – 3 times through

- hanging leg raise	x 11
- full contact twist	x 14
- back extension	x 13

- static stretch

Thursday 2

- warm-up series
- conditioning work

- Tabata intervals – 20 sec. work: 10 sec. rest, done 9 times for each exercise; rest 60 sec. between exercises:	
burpee – DB squat to overhead press – jumping step-up – high-knee run in place	
- stairway walking	x 12 min.
wear a 20–40-lb. weight vest or hold dumbbells; a stair-stepper cardio machine or	
treadmill set to a 5–10 degree incline may be used if you don't have stairs	

- static stretch

Friday 2

- warm-up series
- primary circuit – 8 times through

- BB bent-over row	x 3 (work up to 87.5% 1RM)
- jumping step-up	x 30
- DB snatch	x 4 (use about 25–30% 1RM)
- partner neck work	x 13/each way (do 2 sets in each direction)

- auxiliary circuit – 4 times through

- pull-up	x 11 (or max reps)
- BB shrug	x 11
- tricep pressdown	x 13
- side lunge	x 11/leg

- ab circuit – 3 times through

- V-up	x 13
- DB sidebend	x 11/side
- superman	x 22

- static stretch

Saturday 2 (optional)

- warm-up series
- 22.5 min. jog at moderate pace
- static stretch

Week 3

Monday 3

- warm-up series
- primary circuit - 8 times through

- BB deadlift	x 3 (work up to 90% 1RM)
- jump rope	x 50 hits
- BB jump squat	x 4 (use about 35% 1RM)
- 4-way neck work	x 12/each way (do 2 sets in each direction)

- auxiliary circuit – 4 times through

- BB front lunge	x 10/leg
- leg curl	x 12
- cable pull to face	x 14
- BB triceps extension	x 14

- ab circuit – 3 times through

- straight-leg sit-up	x 10
- standing cable crunch	x 12
- reverse hyper	x 12

- static stretch

Tuesday 3

- warm-up series
- conditioning work

- sled drag forward	x 5 min. (moderate load)
- rest 40 sec.	
- sled drag backward	x 5 min. (moderate load)
- sledgehammer swing circuit	x 5 (40 sec. rest)
perform 10 diagonal left, 10 diagonal right, and 10 straight down on each set	
- medicine ball throw	2 x 5 min. (40 sec. rest)
use a 20–30-lb. ball and throw it as far as you can; jog/walk to it and repeat	
for the entire round; use a variety of throwing techniques	

- static stretch

Wednesday 3

- warm-up series
- primary circuit – 8 times through

- incline bench press	x 3 (work up to 90% 1RM)
- jumping jacks	x 30
- explosive push-up	x 5
- neck bridge	x 14 each way (do 2 sets in each direction)

- auxiliary circuit – 4 times through

- bodyweight dip	x 14
- DB fly	x 14
- glute ham raise	x 12
- BB reverse curl	x 14

- ab circuit – 3 times through

- hanging leg raise	x 11
- full contact twist	x 16
- back extension	x 14

- static stretch

Thursday 3

- warm-up series
- conditioning work

- Tabata intervals – 20 sec. work: 10 sec. rest, done 10 times for each exercise; rest 60 sec. between exercises	
burpee – DB squat to overhead press – jumping step-up – high-knee run in place	
- stairway walking	x 14 min.
wear a 20–40-lb. weight vest or hold dumbbells; a stair-stepper cardio machine or	
treadmill set to a 5–10 degree incline may be used if you don't have stairs	

- static stretch

Friday 3

- warm-up series
- primary circuit – 8 times through

- BB bent-over row	x 3 (work up to 90% 1RM)
- jumping step-up	x 30
- DB snatch	x 4 (use about 35% 1RM)
- partner neck work	x 14/each way (do 2 sets in each direction)

- auxiliary circuit (4 times through)

- pull-up	x 12 (or max reps)
- BB shrug	x 12
- tricep pressdown	x 14
- side lunge	x 12/leg

- ab circuit – 3 times through

- V-up	x 14
- DB sidebend	x 12/side
- superman	x 25

- static stretch

Saturday 3 (optional)

- warm-up series
- 25 min. jog at moderate pace
- static stretch

Week 4

Monday 4

- warm-up series
- primary circuit – 8 times through

- BB deadlift	x 1 (work up to 95% 1RM)
- jump rope	x 50 hits
- BB jump squat	x 4 (use about 35% 1RM)
- 4-way neck work	x 12 each way (do 2 sets in each direction)

- auxiliary circuit – 4 times through

- BB high step-up	x 8/leg
- BB Romanian deadlift	x 10
- BB upright row	x 10
- close grip bench	x 10

- ab circuit – 3 times through

- incline sit-up	x 10
- Russian twist	x 12
- 1-leg reverse hyper	x 10/leg

- static stretch

Tuesday 4

- warm-up series
- conditioning work

- sandbag conditioning circuit	x 5 (60 sec. rest)
use a light sandbag (~25% of bodyweight):	
. shoulder and squat	x 5/side
. clean and press	x 5
. Turkish get-up	x 5/side
. good morning	x 5
- kettlebell conditioning circuit	x 5 (60 sec. rest)
use light kettlebells (15–30 lb.)	
. 1-arm swing (switch hands during upswing)	x 20
. clean and jerk	x 10
. windmill	x 8/side

- static stretch

Wednesday 4

- warm-up series
- primary circuit – 8 times through

- incline bench press	x 1 (work up to 95% 1RM)
- jumping jack	x 30
- MB drop plyo push-up	x 5
- neck bridges w/weight	x 10/each way (do 2 sets in each direction)

- auxiliary circuit – 4 times through

- DB overhead press	x 12
- DB pullover	x 12
- good morning	x 10
- DB hammer curl	x 12

- ab circuit – 3 times through

- twisting incline sit-up	x 12
- Saxon sidebend	x 12
- round back trunk curl	x 14

- static stretch

Thursday 4

- warm-up series
- conditioning work

- 4-corner circuit around basketball court	max trips in 10 min.
. station 1: push-up burpee	x 5
. station 2: step back rubber band pull	x 15
. station 3: vertical jump	x 10
. station 4: mountain climbers	x 30
- rowing machine	3 x 5 min. (60 sec. rest)

- static stretch

Friday 4

- warm-up series
- primary circuit – 8 times through

- BB bent-over row	x 5 (work up to 87.5% 1RM)
- jumping step-up	x 30
- DB snatch	x 4 (use about 35% 1RM)
- partner neck work	x 15 each way (do 2 sets in each direction)

- auxiliary circuit – 4 times through

- lat pull behind neck	x 10
- T-bar shrug	x 12
- French press	x 12
- DB crossover lunge	x 10/leg

- ab circuit – 3 times through

- knee tuck	x 20
- MB torso circle	x 8/direction
- back extension iso hold	3 x 10 sec

- static stretch

Saturday 4 (optional)

- warm-up series
- 25-min. cycling at moderate pace
- static stretch

Week 5

Monday 5

- warm-up series
- primary circuit – 8 times through

- BB deadlift	x 1 (work up to 97.5% 1RM)
- jump rope	x 50 hits
- BB jump squat	x 4 (use about 35% 1RM)
- 4-way neck work	x 12 each way (do 2 sets in each direction)

- auxiliary circuit – 4 times through

- BB high step-ups	x 9/leg
- BB Romanian deadlift	x 11
- BB upright row	x 11
- close grip bench	x 11

- ab circuit – 3 times through

- incline sit-up	x 11
- Russian twist	x 14
- 1-leg reverse hyper	x 12/leg

- static stretch

Tuesday 5

- warm-up series
- conditioning work

- sandbag conditioning circuit	x 5 (50 sec. rest)
use a light sandbag (~25% of bodyweight)	
. shoulder and squat	x 5/side
. clean and press	x 5
. Turkish get-up	x 5/side
. good morning	x 5
- kettlebell conditioning circuit	x 5 (50 sec. rest)
use light kettlebells (15–30 lb.)	
. 1-arm swing (switch hands during upswing)	x 20
. clean and jerk	x 10
. windmill	x 8/side

- static stretch

Wednesday 5

- warm-up series
- primary circuit – 8 times through

- incline bench press	x 1 (work up to 97.5% 1RM)
- jumping jack	x 30
- MB drop plyo push-up	x 5
- neck bridges w/weight	x 10/each way (do 2 sets in each direction)

- auxiliary circuit – 4 times through

- DB overhead press	x 13
- DB pullover	x 13
- good morning	x 11
- DB hammer curl	x 13

- ab circuit – 3 times through

- twisting incline sit-up	x 13
- Saxon sidebend	x 14
- round back trunk curl	x 14

- static stretch

Thursday 5

- warm-up series
- conditioning work

- 4-corner circuit around basketball court	max trips in 12.5 min.
. station 1: push-up burpee	x 5
. station 2: step back rubber band pulls	x 15
. station 3: vertical jumps	x 10
. station 4: mountain climbers	x 30
- rowing machine	3 x 5 min. (50 sec. rest)

- static stretch

Friday 5

- warm-up series
- primary circuit – 8 times through

- BB bent-over row	x 5 (work up to 90% 1RM)
- jumping step-up	x 30
- DB snatch	x 4 (use about 35% 1RM)
- partner neck work	x 15 each way (do 2 sets in each direction)

Friday 5 (cont.)

- auxiliary circuit – 4 times through

- lat pull behind neck	x 11
- T-bar shrug	x 13
- French press	x 13
- DB crossover lunge	x 11/leg

- ab circuit – 3 times through

- knee tuck	x 25
- MB torso circle	x 10/direction
- back extension iso hold	3 x 15 sec

- static stretch

Saturday 5 (optional)

- warm-up series
- 30-min. cycling at moderate pace
- static stretch

Week 6

Monday 6

- warm-up series
- primary circuit – 8 times through

- BB deadlift	x 1 (work up to 100–102.5% 1RM)
- jump rope	x 50 hits
- BB jump squat	x 4 (use about 35% 1RM)
- 4-way neck work	x 12 each way (do 2 sets in each direction)

- auxiliary circuit – 4 times through

- BB high step-up	x 10/leg
- BB Romanian deadlift	x 12
- BB upright row	x 12
- close grip bench	x 12

- ab circuit – 3 times through

- incline sit-up	x 12
- Russian twist	x 16
- 1-leg reverse hyper	x 14/leg

- static stretch

Tuesday 6

- warm-up series
- conditioning work

- sandbag conditioning circuit	x 5 (40 sec. rest)
use a light sandbag (~25% of bodyweight)	
. shoulder and squat	x 5/side
. clean and press	x 5
. Turkish get-up	x 5/side
. good morning	x 5
- kettlebell conditioning circuit	x 5 (40 sec. rest)
use light kettlebells (15–30 lb.)	
. 1-arm swing (switch hands during upswing)	x 20
. clean and jerk	x 10
. windmill	x 8/side

- static stretch

Wednesday 6

- warm-up series
- primary circuit – 8 times through

- incline bench press	x 1 (work up to 100–102.5% 1RM)
- jumping jacks	x 30
- MB drop plyo push-up	x 5
- neck bridges w/weight	x 10 each way (do 2 sets in each direction)

- auxiliary circuit – 4 times through

- DB overhead press	x 14
- DB pullover	x 14
- good morning	x 14
- DB hammer curl	x 14

- ab circuit – 3 times through

- twisting incline sit-up	x 14
- Saxon sidebend	x 16
- round back trunk curl	x 14

- static stretch

Thursday 6

- warm-up series
- conditioning work

- 4-corner circuit around basketball court	max trips in 15 min.
. station 1: push-up burpee	x 5
. station 2: step back rubber band pull	x 15
. station 3: vertical jump	x 10
. station 4: mountain climber	x 30
- rowing machine	3 x 5 min. (40 sec. rest)

- static stretch

Friday 6

- warm-up series
- primary circuit – 8 times through

- BB bent-over row	x 5 (work up to 92.5% 1RM)
- jumping step-up	x 30
- DB snatch	x 4 (use about 35% 1RM)
- partner neck work	x 15/each way (do 2 sets in each direction)

- auxiliary circuit – 4 times through

- lat pull behind neck	x 12
- T-bar shrug	x 14
- French press	x 14
- DB crossover lunge	x 12/leg

- ab circuit – 3 times through

- knee tuck	x 24
- MB torso circle	x 12/direction
- back extension iso hold	3 x 20 sec.

- static stretch

Saturday 6 (optional)

- warm-up series
- 30-min. cycling at moderate pace
- static stretch

Appendix: Conditioning for Combat sports

There are few sports in which the conditioning efforts of past years have been as misguided as in combat athletics. Combat athletics is a general term that includes boxing, kickboxing, wrestling, submission grappling, and any other sport that is based on one-on-one fighting. Coaches and athletes, blindly following tradition, have assumed that the secret to getting fighting fit was logging endless hours of roadwork and staying away from weightlifting to prevent loss of speed. Because these athletes need proper guidance perhaps more than any others, this section presents the collected wisdom of several of top strength and conditioning coaches who specialize in combat athletes.

Article 1

Top Priority! – Conditioning the MMA* & Submission Fighter
by Zach Even-Esh

Have you watched what separates most fighters from the rest of the pack? Yes, a small minority do knock out or tap out their opponents fairly quickly in the opening minute of round one, but this is not the norm. Watch the guys on The *Ultimate Fighter,* all of whom are training to get their shot as a professional in the UFC. In the last fight I watched, one guy was so exhausted after round one that by round two, his hands dropped and he got nailed with a head kick due to fatigue and exhaustion.

A pro athlete should not be in this situation, especially after one round of fighting. The fighter must be optimally prepared for his fights through smart training, not just hard training. I use a variety of tools and methods to improve conditioning. Conditioning is a term I use loosely, as we know that fighters use many different energy systems during a fight or match, so we train using a variety of methods and tools to meet these needs or demands.

Here are some methods we use for conditioning (in addition to actual MMA/grappling training):

- circuits – done for reps, or time
- complexes – done for reps or time
- HIIT (high intensity interval training) – done by monitoring intensity and heart rate, as well as the RPE (rate of perceived exertion) of the athlete

The tools we use are many, allowing us to diversify our conditioning methods listed above:

- sleds
- sandbags
- barbells
- dumbbells
- bodyweight
- kettlebells
- sledgehammers
- ropes
- medicine balls
- logs
- stones

While each truly does work, do not feel the need to use them all: use what works for you, and work hard with the methods I am about to discuss.

One of the easiest ways to improve conditioning, muscular endurance, and lactate toler-ance is through timed circuits. You build up to times that exceed your actual bout times to mentally and physically prepare you to perform past the edge. Later on, I'll discuss tapering so that your body and mind can reap the rewards of your training come fight time as opposed to being burned out or having an accumulation of overuse injuries.

Back to timed circuits: you can use many tools during one circuit or stick to only one method, like bodyweight or free weights. The choice is yours and it depends on factors like available equipment.

Here is a timed circuit that lasts for 5 minutes, with 20 seconds per movement and 10 sec-onds transition time to the next exercise. This schedule means that you will perform two exercises every minute. Having a timer helps, but if you don't have a timer, you can keep it simple and use 10 to 20 reps per set. Keep reps on the lower end if power is the focus and moderate to heavy weights are used, and do higher reps if lighter weights are used and your focus is truly on muscular endurance and lactate tolerance. Circuit training in general is a good way to work on several goals at once, and you can change the focus by changing reps and loads:

- muscular endurance: light weight and high reps (15–20)
- strength endurance: heavy weight and low reps (3–6)
- power endurance: moderate weight and low to moderate reps (3–8)

Here is a sample circuit using a mix of tools. We often do this circuit at a nearby school playground.

Work through the circuit until 10 minutes is complete, quickly going from one movement to the next. At the 5-minute mark, take a brief (30-second) water break (stop the clock) and get back in it for 5 more minutes.

Circuit with variety of tools
- pull-up (vary grip each set) x 6–8 reps
- sandbag Zercher* lunge (alternate forward/reverse/lateral every set) x 6 reps each leg
- parallel bar dips x 10 reps
- leg raises in upright position of dip x 10
- sandbag Zercher* squat x 10 reps
- sandbag burpee plus snatch x 5 reps

*the sandbag is held in the crooks of the arms

You may only be able to perform the above circuit for 3 minutes the first time. Your goal is to progress to two 5-minute rounds, with a short (30-second) break.

The following sandbag complex can be done anywhere. It is convenient because you are only using one tool and waste no time moving to stations or to different exercises. The complex can be done for total time, or until all exercises are performed once for the allotted reps. Never placing the sandbag down for 5 minutes is brutal if you dare to give it a shot! This style of training requires you to drastically lighten the loads until your body improves its lactate tolerance, muscular endurance, and overall conditioning. A 50-lb. bag might be plenty for starters:

Sandbag complex
- clean and press x 6
- push press x 6
- front squat x 6
- Zercher squat jump x 6
- Zercher lunge (any style) x 6 each leg
- bent-over row x 6
- burpee plus push-up plus snatch x 6

The above complex will work lower-body, upper-body and full-body movements together. It's brutal! Try doing 2 to 3 rounds with a work-to-rest ratio of 1:1. As you improve, your rest time can be half of your work time. You can also try to go through the complex twice in a row or go for an extended period of time.

Another way we use a mixture of complexes and time under tension is what I call loaded conditioning: using one training tool, you mix in a movement followed by a carry. Set up a start and finish points A and B anywhere from 25 to 50 feet apart in length.

Loaded conditioning with sandbags
- clean & press x 6
- overhead walk to point B
- front squat in rack position x 6
- rack walk to point A
- bent over row x 6
- hang carry (let the sandbag hang as you grip the sides) to point B
- hang snatch x 6
- Zercher carry to point A

One other method for developing phenomenal conditioning involves technique training mixed with strength training. Do this at your MMA school or possibly the park if you're doing pad work and bodyweight training, but for BJJ* training, do it at the school.

You'll need a sandbag, dumbbell, or kettlebell for each athlete (you can also use body-weight—I prefer tools that take up the least amount of space), or one for every two athletes if you want to break the groups in half. The best way to perform this is for time: 30 seconds seems best, with a 15-second transition period. Be sure to place the training tools away from the edge of the mat, preferably in their own area of use.

You will perform a high-speed technique drill for 30 seconds with a partner and then move to the strength exercise for 30 seconds. This switching back and forth will go on for a minimum of 5 minutes. Optimally, the serious athlete will perform 3 or more rounds.

Here is a sample routine showing high-speed technique drills alternated with kettlebell training:

Technique mixed with strength training
- takedowns with lift x 30 seconds
- 2-hand squats x 30 seconds

- guard passing x 30 seconds (alternate sides)
- snatches from the ground (dead stop, alternate hands every rep) x 30 seconds
- triangles x 30 seconds (alternate sides)
- 2-hand forward or reverse lunges x 30 seconds
- arm bar x 30 seconds (alternate sides)
- 2-hand swing x 30 seconds
- arm bar escapes x 30 seconds (alternate arms)
- hand-to-hand swings x 30 seconds
- mount or side control escapes (alternate sides)

There are so many ways to incorporate conditioning into a fighter's overall regimen. The problem is that not enough time is dedicated to conditioning because too many fighters feel that mat time takes care of all their conditioning needs. This is only part of the puzzle. If you want to be at the top of your game, you must perform variations of conditioning, and the samples provided here are a few ways to ramp up your conditioning.

*MMA = mixed martial arts
*BBJ = Brazilian jiu-jitsu

Zach Even-Esh is a performance coach for combat athletes in New Jersey.
Visit www.combatgrappler.com and www.undergroundstrengthcoach.com to learn more about his methods.

Article 2

A Lesson in Cardiovascular Training
  by Michael Fry

Cardiovascular (adj.): of or pertaining to or involving the heart and blood vessels

Conditioning (n.): to modify so that an act or response previously associated with one stimulus becomes associated with another

Cardiovascular conditioning. It has been called the greatest hold a combat athlete can have, yet so few athletes really have "great" cardiovascular conditioning. I know from my travels that many grapplers feel they already get enough cardio training during their daily training sessions so they do not need to do any on the side. Well, my friends, I am sorry to tell you this but you're wrong.

Before we get started, let's take a look at the definition of conditioning again: *to modify so that an act or response previously associated with one stimulus becomes associated with another*. With that in mind, if we go to practice each and every day of the week and do the same type of training, are we really improving our cardio? The answer is NO.

As you may already know, your body is one of the most advanced machines in the world. Add to that the fact it also has a great memory. Where am I going with this? Follow me for a moment. When we train, our body thinks and it reacts. Did you ever started a new exercise for the first time and have a hard time completing it? Over time, though, this exercise gets easier and that is because of muscle memory. It's really called neuromuscular facilitation, but we will call it muscle memory. The important thing to remember is that cardiovascular training works the same way. It doesn't matter how many hours a day you train, if you're not pushing yourself harder and harder each time (over weeks and months), then sooner or later you are going to get to a point where you just stop improving. The reason for a slowdown is just as the definition stated, "response previously associated with one stimulus becomes associated with another," which means that your body is starting to become conditioned to one way of doing something. It is conditioned to your current training regimen and it needs to be stimulated.

Let's apply this concept to a practical situation that everyone can understand. Did you ever watch two combat athletes go all out for 5 minutes? For most of you, what you will see are two guys who appear to be in fantastic shape ready to pass out. The reason is they have been both training the wrong way and not training hard enough. They might train like animals, but their bodies are used to it and they are not improving.

Let's review. Your body remembers your workouts. It remembers what you did and how hard you did it. When you don't push yourself further than you have before, sooner or later you will reach a point where you are not improving. You want to improve and my goal now is to help you do just that—improve.

Here is a great cardiovascular–muscular endurance program that I want you to do 2 to 3 times a week. Forget about all your benching, squatting, and doing nice arm curls for the next 4 weeks because we are going to create a new stimulus that your body has never felt before. If you do both of these workouts, I promise you that you will see improvements in your cardiovascular and muscular endurance levels that you have never seen before.

The following two workouts are fantastic for combat athletes. I have just used both with members of the Brazilian Top Team, fighters from the UFC and PRIDE, and submission grapplers from all over the world. Here is how it works.

Perform your cardio workout first, and then rest 5 minutes. When you perform this workout, you need to be able to see a watch or clock.

For your weight training, you will be doing a dumbbell clean and press, performing 1 rep every 8 seconds, as shown below in the rest between reps block. Do the workout for 70 seconds, using 40% of your 1RM, and then rest for 75 seconds. Do not put the dumbbell down the entire workout. After you have completed the first set, rest for 75 seconds, then repeat again. Then rest for 5 full minutes.

Now select a dumbbell that is around 20 to 30 pounds and perform the dumbbell complex listed below. Do each exercise one right after another with no rest until the entire cycle is completed. Rest for 2 minutes and repeat 2 to 3 times.

On Wednesday, go to class and ask a teammate to help you with the partner workout. Do this workout as hard as you can for the entire cycle. If you don't you won't improve.

Cardio workout: bike, Airdyne, or Versa-climber
- 15-minute warm-up

Week 1
- Monday & Friday – 10 x 20 sec. work + 10 sec. rest
- Wednesday – 5 x 30 sec. work + 60 sec. rest
                     3 x 20 sec. work + 40 sec. rest
                     2 x 10 sec. work + 30 sec. rest

Week 2
- Monday & Friday – 10 x 20 sec. work + 10 sec. rest
- Wednesday – 5 x 30 sec. work + 60 sec. rest
                     5 x 20 sec. work + 40 sec. rest
                     5 x 10 sec. work + 30 sec. rest

Week 3
- Monday & Friday – 10 x 20 sec. work + 10 sec. rest
- Wednesday – 5 x 30 sec. work + 60 sec. rest
                     5 x 20 sec. work + 40 sec. rest
                     10 x 10 sec. work + 30 sec. rest

Week 4
- Monday – 5 x 30 sec. work + 60 sec. rest
                     5 x 20 sec. work + 40 sec. rest
                     5 x 10 sec. work + 30 sec. rest
- Wednesday – 4 x 30 sec. work + 60 sec. rest
                     6 x 20 sec. work + 40 sec. rest
                     10 x 10 sec. work + 30 sec. rest

Weight training workout – dumbbell clean and press

Week	1	2	3	4	5	6	7	8
Rest between reps	8	8	7	7	6	6	5	5
Set time	70	90	110	130	140	155	165	180
% 1RM	40	40	35	35	35	35	35	35
Sets	2	2	2	2	2	2	2	2
Rest between sets	75	65	55	50	45	40	30	20

Rest 5 minutes.

Dumbbell complex

- DB hammer curls .... x 6
- DB upright row .... x 6
- DB high pull snatch regular .... x 6
- DB parallel press .... x 6
- DB bent-over row .... x 6
- DB rotational squat push press .... x 6
- DB alternate leg lunges (front to back) .... x 6 + 6
- DB alternate leg lunges (left to right) .... x 6 + 6
- DB squat upright row .... x 6
- DB clean & press .... x 12

Rest for 2 minutes and repeat 3 times.

Wednesday – Partner Workout

Training with your partner can be done at Brazilian jiu-jitsu school or on gym mats. Perform 3 sets x 1–2 minutes rest. Add 15 seconds each week to time.

1. Pummel – 30 seconds (fighting for inside control)
2. Sprawl to double leg partner lifts – 30 seconds
3. High knees from the clinch to the armpit – 30 seconds (alternate left and right)
4. Pummeling – 30 seconds
5. Lift and dump (bear hug to single leg/high crotch lift, take to the mat) – 30 seconds
6. Lift and return to the mat (wrestling stand-up) – 30 seconds
7. Pummeling – 30 seconds
8. Sprawl to partner lift – 30 seconds
9. Pummeling – 60 seconds
10. Partner carries – 60 seconds

Enjoy, improve, and become a champion.

Michael Fry is the owner of Grappler's Gym and www.grapplersgym.com and the author of *The Grappler's Guide to Sports Nutrition*.

Article 3

MaxCondition Endurance Training
by Jamie Hale

As with all other modes of MaxCondition training, protocols to enhance work capacity vary among athletes. In general, my athletes do not dedicate a great deal of time to low-intensity extensive aerobic training (e.g., running 5 miles, biking for 1 hour). If they are endurance athletes (cross-country, marathoners, distance kayakers, etc.), this protocol changes as they need more aerobic activity. If an athlete who has had no experience with endurance training comes to me, I will probably advise low-intensity aerobic training for 3 to 4 weeks (1.5 to 2 miles), 3 to 4 days per week. After this period of forming an aerobic base, work will become more intense and specific in nature. I like to introduce the athlete to aerobic–anaerobic interval training along with non-weighted and weighted GPP.

In a typical aerobic–anaerobic interval session, my athletes simply alternate between low- to moderate-intensity aerobic activity and high-intensity anaerobic activity.

Aerobic–anaerobic interval training

- movement performed on a rowing machine or bike: moderate activity for 2 minutes followed by 10 seconds of max effort sprinting; perform for 7–10 cycles

- movement performed on a heavy bag: punch heavy bag at a moderate pace for 1 minute followed by 1 minute of max effort punch output. Repeat the cycle 10 times; total duration of exercise is 10 minutes. This exercise teaches the athlete to make the transition from primarily aerobic activity to anaerobic activity

Lactate threshold and anaerobic threshold training are also used frequently in my programs as they are an important determinant in an athlete's work capabilities. Keep in mind that no matter what an athlete's VO2 max is, if the lactate threshold is low, this oxygen cannot be utilized.

Lactate threshold and anaerobic threshold training

- punch out drills: punch a heavy bag non-stop for 1 to 1.5 minutes; throw straining punches with no pause between strikes. Perform 3 rounds, resting 30 to 45 seconds between rounds

Jamie Hale is a sports conditioning coach, author, gym owner, and fitness and nutrition consultant. Learn more about his methods at www.maxcondition.com.

Online Resources

Part of being an informed coach or athlete is gathering information and ideas from many different sources. Fortunately the Internet allows you to access a lot of valuable information with just a few keystrokes. The following is a short list of some of the more valuable online training sites.

Crossfit – www.crossfit.com

Crossfit is a website and set of affiliated gyms that focus on blending strength, conditioning, and general athleticism. Their workouts feature Olympic weightlifting, gymnastic exercises, climbing, and a wide variety of other modes. The Crossfit training system provides a perfect example of how to develop strength and endurance simultaneously while changing the workouts often to prevent boredom and burnout. The website includes a daily workout and a forum that allows you to ask questions and compare your performance to others who complete the same workout.

Elite Fitness Systems – www.elitefts.com

Elite FTS is a site run by Dave Tate and a crew of serious powerlifters and strength athletes. They have question and answer forums so that you can get information on powerlifting, general strength and conditioning, and sports specific training. There is a lot of discussion about building GPP by dragging sleds, using sledgehammers, etc. Martin Rooney, author of the *Warrior Training* book and DVD set, also answers many of the questions on the forums.

Maxcondition – www.maxcondition.com

Maxcondition is a site run by top strength and conditioning coach Jamie Hale. Numerous articles cover such topics as sports nutrition and fat loss, lifting and strength training, high-intensity interval training, flexibility, and abdominal training. Maxcondition also has a forum so you can discuss or post questions on anything related to training. The site is a great resource for coaches and athletes.

Underground Strength Coach – www.undergroundstrengthcoach.com

Underground Strength Coach is a site run by Zach Even-Esh and is devoted to innovative strength and conditioning work using a variety of training methods. There are articles on sandbags, kettlebells, strongman training, and workouts that incorporate modalities you've probably never heard of. The site also has a forum where you can ask questions and discuss training with knowledgeable professionals.

ExRx.net – www.exrx.net

ExRx is one of the most information-dense websites on strength, conditioning, and fitness on the web. It contains information on all aspects of health and fitness. ExRx has a number of very useful caloric requirement and body fat calculators if you need help with your nutritional program. You can also use other calculators to find the metabolic cost of different activities or how you rank on different fitness tests compared to the average American. There is an exercise database with descriptions and animations of hundreds of different lifts and an extensive links list for further research.

T-Nation – www.t-nation.com

T-Nation is an online magazine and discussion forum with a lot of good, informative training articles each month. Topics range from strength training to bodybuilding to sport-specific conditioning. In addition, there is a forum attached to the end of each article so that you can discuss it with other readers and the author. All of the previously published articles are archived so that you can find any you might have missed. Highly recommended.

Grappler's Gym – www.grapplersgym.com

The Grappler's Gym is a training site devoted to wrestling and other grappling arts. Despite the sport-specific focus, there are numerous training articles on strength–endurance and high-intensity conditioning that can benefit any athlete. There are also articles on nutrition, weight control, and health and first aid issues common to many different combat and contact sports. Even if you don't wrestle, you will find valuable training information to help you get in the best shape of your life.

REFERENCES

Baechle, T. R., ed. *Essentials of Strength and Conditioning*. Human Kinetics. 1994.

Brookfield, J. Formula for Success. *MILO*. 10(2):55-57. 2002.

Brookfield, J. *Training with Cables for Strength*. IronMind. 2001.

Brooks, G. A., T. D. Fahey, and T. P. White. *Exercise Physiology: Human Bioenergetics and Its Applications*. Mayfield. 1996.

Chen, M. J., X. Fan, and S. T. Moe. Criterion-related validity of the Borg ratings of perceived exertion scale in healthy individuals: a meta-analysis. *J. Sport Sci*. 20(11):873-899. 2002.

Csikszentmihalyi, M. *Flow: The Psychology of Optimal Experience*. Harper. 1991.

Fischer, W. *SCRAPPER Bodyweight Conditioning Mod.1* 2003.

Fox, E. L and D. K. Matthews. *Interval Training: Conditioning for Sports and General Fitness*. W. B. Saunders. 1974.

Furey, M. *Combat Conditioning: Functional Exercises for Fitness and Combat Sports*. 1998.

Hale, J. *Maxcondition*. 2004.

Heyward, V. H. *Advanced Fitness Assessment & Exercise Prescription* 3rd ed. Human Kinetics. 1998.

Ishikawa, T. and D. Draeger. *Judo Training Methods*. Tuttle. 1999

Javorek, I. *Javorek "Complex" Conditioning*. 2004.

Jeffries, B. *Super Strength and Endurance for Martial Arts*. 2005.

Jeffries, B. *Twisted Conditioning*. 2004.

Jeffries, B. *Twisted Conditioning II*. 2005.

Jesse, J. *Wrestling Physical Conditioning Encyclopedia*. Athletic Press. 1974.

Johnson, D. A. *Wrestling Drill Book*. Leisure Press.1991

Johnson, B. *Bodyweight Exercises for Extraordinary Strength*. IronMind. 2005.

Jones, B. *The Complete Sandbag Training Course*. IronMind. 2004.

Kahn, A. H. *The Speed Bag Bible*. Rehabilitation & Sports Consulting. 1995.

Karlsson, Jan. *Antioxidants and Exercise*. Human Kinetics. 1997.

McCallum, J. *The Complete Keys To Progress*. IronMind. 1993.

Morgan, R. E. and G. T. Adamson. *Circuit Training*. G. Bell and Sons. 1959

Noakes, T. D. *The Lore of Running*. 3rd ed. Human Kinetics. 1991.

Rooney, M. *Training for Warriors: The Team Renzo Gracie Workout* (Book and DVDs). 2004.

Santana, J. C. *The Essence of Band and Pulley Training* (DVD and Companion Guide). IHP. 2005.

Santana, J. C. *The Essence of Bodyweight Training* (DVD and Companion Guide). IHP. 2005.

Santana, J. C. *The Essence of Medicine Ball Training* (DVD and Companion Guide). IHP. 2005.

Santana, J. C. and R. Ferguson. *S.A.I.D. Training: For Gi-Grappling* DVD. Intocombat. 2006.

Santana, J. C. and R. Ferguson. *S.A.I.D. Training: For Mixed Martial Arts* DVD. Intocombat. 2006.

Santana, J. C. and R. Ferguson. *S.A.I.D. Training: For No-gi Grappling* DVD. *Intocombat*. 2006.

Schwartz, L. *Heavyhands: The Ultimate Exercise*. Warner Books. 1982.

Siff, Mel C. *Supertraining*. Supertraining Institute. 2003.

Sonnon, S. *Clubbell Training for Circular Strength: An Ancient Tool for the Modern Athlete*. RMAX. 2003.

Strossen, R. *SUPER SQUATS: How to Gain 30 Pounds of Muscle in 6 Weeks*. IronMind. 1989.

Tabata, I., K. Nishimura, M. Kouzaki, et al. Effects of moderate intensity endurance and high intensity intermittent training on anaerobic capacity and VO_2 max. *Med. Sci. Sports Exerc*. 28:1327-1330. 1996.

Tsatsouline, P. *The Naked Warrior*. Dragon Door. 2003.

Tsatsouline, P. *The Russian Kettlebell Challenge*. Dragon Door. 2001.

Yoshioka, M., E. Doucet, S. St-Pierre, et al. Impact of high-intensity exercise on energy expenditure, lipid oxidation, and body fatness. *Int. J. Obesity*. 25:332-339. 2001.

INDEX

Adamson, G.T. 40, 42–43
adaptations 22–24, 27–28
    central 22–23
    peripheral 22–23
    psychological 24
adenine diphosphate (ADP) 16
adenosine triphosphate (ATP) 16–17, 20
agility work 76–78
    agility ladder 81

bioenergetics 16
body recomposition 24
    body fat 24–25
bodyweight exercises 85–92
Borg, Gunnar 56
boxing, kickboxing routines 151–152

cable/band training 114–115
cheat repetitions 46
circuit training 40–41, 59–60
combat training 96–103, 192–205
cool-down 34–35
core training 123–129
    core workouts 155
creatine phosphate (CP) 16–17, 19–20
Csikszentmihlayi, Mihaly 130
    flow 130

deck of cards routine 157–158
delayed onset muscle soreness (DOMS) 39, 61, 105, 118
density 29
detraining 29
drop sets 46

energy pathways 16
environmental factors 132–133
excess post-exercise oxygen consumption (EPOC) 25
exercise mode 30, 51

fartlek running 52
fast twitch (Type II) fibers 19, 49, 92
fatigue 19, 21, 24
    general 40
    specific 40
finishers 53–54
forced repetitions 46
free weights 118–122
    circuits 134–137
    complexes 138–139
frequency 30
Furey, Matt 157

general adaptation syndrome (GAS) 64
general physical preparation (GPP) 12–15
glucose 16–17
glycogen 16–17, 21, 23
glycolysis 17–19, 23
glycolytic system 16–17, 20, 22, 48
grappling 100–103

heart rate 58–59
heavybags 73–76
Heavyhands 153
homeostasis 27
hydration 39
hypertrophy training 45–46

intensity 30–31, 51, 56
interval training 49–51
    interval duration 49
    Tabata 52
    timers 53
    training progression 143–144

Javorek, Istvan 121
jumping 78–80
jumping rope 116–118
    routines 141

kata workouts 152
kettlebell training 110–113

lactate threshold 18–19, 21
lactic acid 16–20, 23–24, 40, 48–50, 57, 61
law enforcement training 146–149
Lee, Buddy 117

macronutrients 37–38
maximal cardiac output 18
maximal stroke volume 18
medicine balls 71–73
micronutrients 38–39
mindfulness meditation 131
Morgan, R.E. 40, 42–43
mouthpieces 69

needs analysis 66–68
nutrition 36–39

obstacle course 147–149
100 reps routine 144–145
overload 27–28
overtraining 45, 53, 64–65
oxidative system 16–17, 20–22
oxygen extraction 18

peripheral heart action (PHA) 46–47
phosphagen system 16, 19–20, 22, 48
physiology 12, 16
programming 26
progression 27, 51
psychology 130–132
pyramid workouts 142–143